SURGERY

George Crile, Jr., M.D.
SURGERY

Your Choices
Your Alternatives

A Merloyd Lawrence Book
DELACORTE PRESS/SEYMOUR LAWRENCE

A *Merloyd Lawrence* Book
Published by
Delacorte Press/Seymour Lawrence
1 Dag Hammarskjold Plaza
New York, N.Y. 10017

Sections of Chapters 6, 7, 8, 10, and 11 were previously published in somewhat different form. Grateful acknowledgment is made to the following:

American Medical News: "A Way to Identify Inappropriate Surgery" (February 16, 1976).

Harper's Magazine: "The Surgeon's Dilemma" Copyright © 1975 by *Harper's Magazine.* All rights reserved. Reprinted from the May 1975 issue by special permission.

Hospital Physician: "Kicking the Fee-for-Service Habit" (October 1975).

Medical World News: "On the Other Hand" reprinted from *Medical World News.* Copyright © 1977 by McGraw-Hill, Inc.

Modern Medicine: "Somebody Do Something" column (June 15, 1977), "Miracles of Medicine: Do They Help People or Glorify Technocracy?" (February 15, 1977), and "RX for American Medicine: The Best of Both Worlds" (August 15, 1977).

Copyright©1978 by George Crile, Jr.

All rights reserved. No part of this book may be reproduced or transmitted in any form or by any means, electronic or mechanical, including photocopying, recording, or by any information storage and retrieval system, without the written permission of the Publisher, except where permitted by law.

Manufactured in the United States of America

First printing

Designed by Laura Bernay

Library of Congress Cataloging in Publication Data

Crile, George, 1907–
  Surgery.

  "A Merloyd Lawrence book."
  Includes index.
  1. Surgery—Popular works. 2. Surgery—Decision making. I. Title. [DNLM: 1. Surgery—Popular works. WQ100.3 C929s]
  RD31.3.C74   617   78–19020
  ISBN 0–440–07715–X

Acknowledgments

I am grateful to my colleagues at the Cleveland Clinic for their advice and help in editing the sections that pertained to each of their specialties.

I am also grateful to Merloyd Lawrence for her detailed and knowledgeable editing of the manuscript.

Finally, I am indebted to Dr. Arthur Ulene, who made helpful suggestions in the many areas of his broad field of medical knowledge.

To
Katharine Murphy Crile,
whose father encouraged me
to write along these lines.

Contents

Foreword xiii

PART ONE: Choices in Surgical Care

I   The Way It Was 3

II An Example of Controversy:
Diagnosis and Treatment of Cancer of the
Breast 8
>Mammography—When and How Often?/9
Biopsy—When and How?/10
Surgery—How Radical?/13
Radiation—In Which Cases?/24
Endocrine Therapy—Surgical or Medical?/25

Contents

Chemotherapy—An Open Question/28
Scans—When Are They Useful?/30
How to Choose and Who Should Choose/31

III   Controversy in Other Types of Cancer   . . 33

Cancer in Situ of the Cervix/34
Cancer of the Head and Neck/37
Cancer of the Larynx/39
Cancer of the Lung/41
Melanomas/43
Cancer of the Pancreas/46
Cancer of the Prostate Gland/48
Small, Low-lying Cancers of the Rectum/52
Cancers of the Skin/59
Cancer of the Thyroid/60
General Considerations/64

IV   Choices in Nonmalignant Disease   66

Appendicitis/66
Arthritis/67
Back Pain/68
Duodenal Ulcer/69
Gallstones/73
Goiter/76
Heart Disease (Coronary Bypass Surgery)/82
Hemorrhoids/83
Hernia Repair/85
Hyperthyroidism/86
Ingrown Toenails/89
Lipomas/90
Pilonidal Cyst or Sinus/90
Polyps/93
Prostate Gland—Benign Enlargement/95
Tonsillectomy and Adenoidectomy/97
Vaginal Repair Operations/98
Varicose Veins/99
Vascular Surgery/100

V   Annual Checkup and the
Diagnosis of Surgical Problems   102

The Complete Physical/103
Laboratory Tests/108

CONTENTS

PART TWO: Surgical Care and Our Medical System

VI	Fee-for-Service Surgery	113
VII	Surgery Under State Medicine, Prepaid Health Plans (HMO), and Fee-for-Service	127
VIII	Inappropriate Operations and How to Eliminate Them	132
IX	Informed Consent	141
X	Public Education About Health	146
XI	The Law of Diminishing Returns	151
	Notes	162
	Index	169

[xi]

Foreword

When surgeons don't agree on what the best treatment is, how can a patient decide which of several alternatives to accept?

There is no answer to this question, because there is no "best" treatment. For example, are we speaking of best in terms of eradicating the disease, of best in terms of the safety of the patient, of best in terms of the comfort of the patient —or of what is best for the surgeon, in terms of safety from malpractice suits, the size of fee, or of the time and trouble required to perform the operation?

Even in cases in which there is no agreement among surgeons as to the best treatment for a disease, there still may be clear and formidable differences between treatments in terms of the *survival* of the patient and of the comfort and quality of his or her life. This is because some surgeons view

Foreword

certain diseases the way the clergy of the Middle Ages viewed the Devil—as something to be exorcised regardless of the consequences to the person. It is also why so many of the most bitter controversies are about the treatment of cancer.

This book has been written to make patients aware of legitimate differences in opinion among the best-qualified surgeons. I would like to enable and encourage patients to ask such questions as, "What are the alternatives to operation, Doctor? Can I be treated by medicine? Can I be treated by radiation therapy? Are there other less extensive, less deforming, and less painful operations than the one you suggested? What is the mortality rate of the operation (the chance of my dying as a result of it)—both nationally, and in the hospital in which you suggest that I have the operation? How many of these operations do you yourself do each year?" These and other probing questions may lead to the adoption of a method of treatment other than the one originally proposed or may result in referral to a specialist who is better qualified to treat the disease. If so, the treatment finally agreed on may be more effective or safer and with fewer side effects than the one originally suggested.

Many patients are fearful of asking questions, being afraid their physicians might construe them as showing a lack of confidence. Perhaps a decade ago this might have been a valid fear, for it is only in recent years that emphasis has been laid, both medically and legally, on the necessity of the patient's giving his or her informed consent to any suggested treatment. This cannot be done without a frank discussion of the risks and benefits of treatment and of the qualifications of the physicians and surgeons who will give it. For these reasons patients should never hesitate to speak openly of what is in their minds.

The principles of surgical treatment are relatively simple. They can be explained either in clear English or by analogy.

Foreword

If you, the patient, insist that your doctor explain why the suggested treatments should be given and what alternatives to surgery there are, you will be able to enter into the final decisions and participate actively in protecting your own best interests. A person's body is his or her own, and it is you, the patient, not the doctor, who has the final say about how that body will be treated.

The perspective from which this book is written is that of a surgeon. I was brought up in a family dominated by the vivid personality of a surgeon, my world-famous father. I have no remembrance of ever wanting to become anything other than a surgeon. My entire professional career, from which I am now retired, has been devoted to the practice and to the teaching of surgery and to research in surgery and allied fields. Yet my dominant interest has never been in surgery itself. It has been in biology and in the various ways in which knowledge of science can affect and direct the treatment of disease.

Surgery is one of the most effective ways of influencing the course of disease, but, as is the case with most other treatments, it is a double-edged sword. It can affect the course of a disease either for better or for worse. Moreover, the side effects and complications of surgery are prompt and often irreversible, and its immediate mortality is higher than that of most other treatments. That is why surgery is the most dramatic branch of medicine and why patients quite rightly have an innate fear of operations. It is also why patients facing surgery have both the right and the responsibility to ask questions.

These questions are not easily answered, because for many diseases there is no agreement, even among surgeons and other experts in the field of health, about what constitutes the best treatment. In 1976, for example, a 713-page textbook of surgery entitled *Controversy in Surgery* was pub-

FOREWORD

lished.[1] In each of the thirty surgically treatable diseases that were discussed, there were two or more conflicting opinions as to how the disease should be treated—surgically, by radical operations, or by conservative operations; medically; or by radiation therapy.

One of the factors that enters into these decisions is the patient himself—his age, his temperament, his ambitions, and his phobias. I suggest that no two patients have the same needs. I also suggest that because of these differences the best treatment for one person is not necessarily the best for another. Finally, I suggest that the patient should enter into the dialogue that decides what treatment will be given.

The first half of this book is designed to spell out the choices of operations and the alternatives to surgery and to help the patient select the one most appropriate for his or her individual needs. Part Two considers the background against which both patient and doctor make their decisions. It discusses the potential conflict of interest in the fee-for-service system of paying the surgeon. Finally, it takes up various ways, including public education about health, in which the government, the medical profession, and the citizen can improve the context in which health decisions are made.

It is my hope that this book will be useful to patients for whom operations have been advised. The patient can and should become an intelligent participant in discussions about surgery. A better decision will be made if the patient is informed about the disease and knows something of the choices and alternatives that are available for its treatment.

There are choices.
There are alternatives.
It is up to you, the patient, to learn about them.

PART ONE

Choices in Surgical Care

I

The Way It Was

Forty-four years ago, when I finished medical school, the art and science of surgery was written in LARGE BLACK LETTERS that both doctors and patients could read. The message said "THAT IS THE DIAGNOSIS" and "THIS IS THE TREATMENT." It was all so simple then.

I remember forty years ago, when I was a resident in a hospital where the chief of surgery was noted for his charm and manners. A distinguished lady had been operated on for a cancer of the rectum. All of the rectum and lower bowel had been removed and a colostomy established. For ten days the woman was desperately ill and nearly died. Finally she regained consciousness and was able to talk. On rounds the chief came by to see her. She asked him trustfully, "Do you think you got all my hemorrhoids so they'll never come back?"

CHOICES IN SURGICAL CARE

If a woman had a cancer of the breast, both she and her surgeon knew that she must have a radical mastectomy. The technique was standardized and known to all. Explanations and discussions were superfluous. "If the biopsy shows cancer, we will go right ahead and take care of it," was all the surgeon said. No one thought of getting a signed permission.

For the thirty diseases mentioned in the Foreword, those about whose treatment surgeons now disagree, surgeons in the 1930s not only agreed which were best treated by surgery but agreed also about what operation was best. Treatment of cancer is one of the best examples. In the 1930s radiation therapy for the treatment of cancer had not yet been developed to the point of being competitive with surgery. Chemotherapy had not even been thought of. Patients had confidence in what their doctors told them. They did not read in women's magazines or hear on television all about the latest type of treatment. They did not run off to Mexico to take Laetrile.

In the period of which I am writing, the surgical profession was standing poised and ready to leap into three decades of ever more radical techniques. Already the Halsted radical mastectomy (see Chapter 2) was almost universally accepted; many surgeons were performing radical dissections for cancers in the neck (see Chapter 3), and those who had learned how were doing the radical operation for rectal cancer (see Chapter 3). But that was about the extent of radical surgery. The chest had not yet been invaded nor the heart violated. But then, in rapid succession, came sulfanilamide and the antibiotics to control infections. Intravenous barbiturates and relaxants rapidly replaced chloroform and ether as anesthetic agents. Postoperative complications were greatly reduced, making it safer to perform longer and more intricate operations. Shock was avoided by more liberal use of intravenous fluids. Blood banks were organized. Diagnosis of cancer

The Way
It Was

by examining a frozen section under the microscope, while the patient was still in the operating room, became routine. The use of *cytology* (the study of individual cells or groups of cells as in the Papanicolaou test, or *Pap smear*) enabled many cancers to be diagnosed earlier than ever before. General practitioners stopped giving anesthesia. Gradually the nurse anesthetist was replaced by the physician anesthesiologist or worked under his or her supervision. Anesthesiologists were trained and specialized in anesthesia. Under their direction the basic principles of physiology were transplanted from unopened textbooks to the recovery room.

Thinking back to the 1930s, it seems strange that Dr. Wangensteen had not yet popularized the gastric suction apparatus, later used routinely to draw off excess fluid and gas from overdistended stomachs and intestines. *Intubation* of the trachea—putting a tube into the windpipe to facilitate breathing—was scarcely practiced at all when I started my residency. Antibiotics had not been dreamed of. Small wonder that in those days ultraradical operations were not done. The patients could not have survived them.

As the science of surgery progressed, so did its techniques, expanding into the performance of ever more radical operations, especially in cancer surgery. At that time it was not yet known that even early in the course of the disease, the type of cancer that can *metastasize* (i.e., spread from the points of origin to other places in the body) can invade the blood vessels and shed cells into the bloodstream with the result that the cells are carried by the moving blood to lungs, liver, or elsewhere. Whether these cells live, reproduce, and give rise to *metastases* (new cancerous growths) depends on the conditions they meet where they come to rest and on the vigilance of the white cells which constitute the patient's chief defense. But it was not until the 1950s that, thanks to the skill that pathologists had developed in recognizing can-

CHOICES IN
SURGICAL CARE

cer cells on Pap smears, it was possible to recognize cancer cells in the blood of the veins that drained the cancers.

After the discovery of cancer cells in blood, scientists began to look on the spread of cancer in a totally different light. Prior to the demonstration of cancer cells in the blood, it had been assumed (for no obvious reason) that cancers started out localized and therefore would be curable simply by removing them. It was assumed that later on they spread to the regional lymph nodes, such as, in the case of cancer of a breast, those of the armpit. Finally, it was thought that, after residing in the nodes for some time, the cancer spread into the bloodstream and was carried to distant organs. This was the simplistic theory that, in the 1940s, prompted surgeons to perform ever more radical operations.

The regional lymph nodes were assumed to be the key to the cancer's attack on the body. In the name of removing the last cancer cell in the last lymph node, the scope of operations was steadily increased until in some cases the operations designed to remove the nodes became more dangerous than leaving the nodes alone. At that time little consideration was given to the *morbidity* (deformity, disability, and discomfort) inflicted by ultraradical operations.

That was the situation in the 1950s, when the basic principles of the spread of cancer began to be understood. At last scientists began to see that local treatments, no matter how extensive or how mutilating, could not cure a cancer that already had spread to distant organs. It was at this point that the disagreements about treatment began. Surgeons oriented to traditional beliefs continued to perform operations that were progressively more radical. Others, who had adopted the point of view that extreme expansion of local treatment could not increase survival, were opposed to ultraradical surgery. They recognized the dangers of the radical operations, and they believed that the lives and welfare

The Way It Was

of patients were being sacrificed in order to satisfy a vain hope of cure.

Other conditions treatable by surgery, such as duodenal ulcer, heart disease, circulatory disorders, and advanced arthritis, have seen the rise of equally elaborate and radical techniques. For these conditions, too, questions are now being asked about the appropriateness, safety, and effect on life expectancy of particular surgical treatments.

The type of treatment accepted can make an enormous difference, both in survival and in morbidity. These differences depend not only on what treatment is given but also on who gives it. That is what makes it hard for the patient, because if he or she does not ask the right questions, there is no way to determine what the risks are or whether there are alternatives. In this discussion of risk we are not much concerned with common operations that have clear indications, such as removal of the gallbladder for gallstones that are giving pain, or removal of a fibroid uterus for excessive and uncontrollable bleeding. We are particularly concerned with the relatively less frequent operations, which have less clear indications, and which, to be done safely, require some degree of specialization. We also are vitally concerned with diseases like cancer of the breast that are both serious and common, and whose treatment is at present clouded in controversy.

II

An Example of Controversy: Diagnosis and Treatment of Cancer of the Breast

In November 1976 the National Cancer Institute, the American Cancer Society, and the White House sponsored an international meeting entitled "Breast Cancer: A Report to the Profession."[1] Leading clinicians and scientists from Great Britain, other parts of Europe, and North America spoke for two days on all aspects of the disease, but chiefly on its diagnosis and treatment. At the end of the last day only one fact was apparent: Among the world's authorities there was no agreement about either diagnosis or treatment.

An Example of Controversy:
Diagnosis and Treatment of Cancer of the Breast

Mammography—When and How Often?

At the meeting just mentioned a respected scientist from the National Institutes of Health warned that *mammograms* (x-rays of the breast) used to screen population groups exposed the breast to radiation and thereby ran the risk of inducing cancer. He spoke of studies suggesting that this was particularly true in women who, because of personal or family history, were thought to be at increased risk. A small amount of radiation given to these predisposed women might trigger the development of cancer. Not until a woman was beyond the age of fifty, when the mammograms were more effective in showing small tumors and when the risk of inducing a cancer by radiation was decreased, could any gain in survival be expected from having annual x-rays of the breast. He concluded that if the breasts were x-rayed annually from age thirty-five on, there might be more years of life lost from cancers induced by radiation than gained from finding cancers when they were small and curable. However, neither he nor anyone else questioned the use of mammography when there were symptoms or signs of an abnormality in the breast.

A number of other speakers immediately rose to defend mammography. They pointed out its many advantages in the early detection of breast cancer and showed that they had been able to reduce the dose of radiation given by a mammogram to a small fraction of what it had been before.

Obviously there is a middle ground that is best, but exactly where this lies has not yet been determined. In such a case the patient's judgment is as good as the doctor's. My personal opinion is that unless there is a special reason for it, mammography should not be used until the age of forty. A second

CHOICES IN
SURGICAL CARE

mammogram at forty-five and a third at fifty would be acceptable. After that a mammogram every two or three years should give protection without significant danger.

The above discussion applies only to the use of mammography in the screening of population groups, not to its use in helping to diagnose a known lump or mass. In such cases the small risk of radiation is far outweighed by its benefits.

Biopsy—When and How?

If you have a lump in your breast and consult a surgeon, he may, in the office, freeze the skin to anesthetize it and put a needle into the lump. If it is a cyst, he will withdraw the fluid and you are cured. No further treatment is necessary. If there is no fluid, the surgeon may suck up a little of the tissue juice, spread it out on a slide like a Pap smear, and send it to the pathologist to see if there are any cancer cells in it. This is known as an *aspiration biopsy*. If there are abnormal-looking cells, there is a 95 percent chance that this is a true cancer and that an operation will be necessary. All of this is discussed with you, and if there is any doubt about the clinical, x-ray, or pathological diagnosis, you are admitted to the hospital for confirmation of the diagnosis by biopsy and frozen section. If there is no doubt, or if frozen section confirms the diagnosis made on the smear, the surgeon proceeds with the operation that has been agreed upon.

If the pathologist interprets the smear as negative, showing no cancer cells, there is a 95 percent chance that no cancer is present. But to be sure about the other 5 percent, the surgeon will advise removal of the lump. Since the odds

An Example of Controversy: Diagnosis and Treatment of Cancer of the Breast

are so strong against the lump being malignant, no plans are made for performing a cancer-type operation. An *open biopsy* (i.e., an incision made and tissue removed for analysis) will be done in the operating room of the hospital, generally on an outpatient basis. If the pathologist finds no cancer in the lump, no further treatment is necessary.

In the unlikely event that in spite of the negative aspiration biopsy the pathologist finds a cancer whose cells had not appeared on the smear, the surgeon will arrange with you to enter the hospital at a later date and will discuss with you the type of operation that he proposes to do. There is no hurry about this operation because the lump is out. Countless studies have shown that the cancer is not spread by there being a reasonable delay between a biopsy which removes the tumor and the definitive operation.[2] Some surgeons even believe that it is better to excise the cancer before doing a more extensive operation, because it cuts down on the chances of there being cancer cells in blood and lymphatic vessels that might be implanted in the wound and give rise to local recurrences.

The great advantage of the step-by-step diagnosis, with separation of the biopsy from the definitive operation, is that the patient is not threatened with loss of the breast unless, or at least until, the diagnosis has been definitely established. Let us consider what happens if the surgeon takes the other course, the one which until recently most surgeons have followed.

The surgeon informs you that the lump in your breast may be malignant. He makes no attempt to diagnose it in the office or to aspirate it, even if it is a cyst. He admits you to the hospital and orders all the costly tests that are necessary in case the tumor is malignant and a major operation is to be done. You sign permission either for the surgeon to do whatever operation he thinks best, or more often, today, for a

CHOICES IN SURGICAL CARE

radical or modified radical mastectomy to be performed if the biopsy shows cancer. You are anesthetized, not knowing whether you will wake up minus a breast. If the lump is a simple cyst the biopsy has been totally unnecessary because it could have been cured by aspiration. In about four cases out of five (in some hospitals in as many as seven out of eight) such biopsies show no cancer. The expensive preoperative tests and hospitalization, and the fear of mastectomy, all have been needless. The procedure could have been carried out just as well without admitting the patient to the hospital and without having frightened her about the treatment.

In the last three years many surgeons have moved away from the second method of doing breast biopsies. More and more they are separating the biopsy and the definitive procedure. Many, however, still refuse to accept the massive evidence that there is no harm in separating the biopsy from the operation. Many even refuse to aspirate cysts, in spite of the fact that the safety and efficacy of aspiration has been known for more than fifty years.

The most important reason for separating the biopsy and the definitive operation occurs in cases in which the cancer is small and upon physical and x-ray examination does not appear to be definitely malignant. In some such cases it may be difficult for the pathologist who examines the tissue under the microscope to tell whether or not it is a true cancer. This is particularly true if the pathologist has to rely on a quickly cut frozen section, which does not give as good detail as the final sections that usually take twenty-four hours to process. Mistakes are possible even on the permanent sections, but are much more apt to be made on frozen section.

Surgeons, like any skilled artisans who have mastered a technique, are creatures of habit. Having once persuaded themselves of the advantages of a certain method of treatment, they are not apt to change, especially when a needle

An Example of Controversy: Diagnosis and Treatment of Cancer of the Breast

biopsy or aspiration of a cyst in the office commands a fee of about $20 compared to $100 to $200 or more for an open biopsy. I do not imply that in the minds of most surgeons the fee is a conscious consideration. Yet I believe that if the economics were reversed and surgeons were paid $200 for the office treatment and only $20 for an open biopsy, over a period of years there would be a higher proportion of breast cysts treated in the office.

We have seen that there are at least four alternative methods of establishing a diagnosis. Some entail hospitalization, increased expense, and increased fear. Others entail none of these disadvantages. The important thing for you is to know of the alternatives and to ask about them. But these are only the beginnings of the breast-cancer controversy.

Surgery—How Radical?

Much more violent and, from the patient's standpoint, a much more important controversy surrounds the decision as to how a cancer will be treated. I am not going to go into this in great detail, because a number of books are available on the subject.[3] Suffice it to say that there is no proven "best" treatment for cancer of the breast.

This became perfectly clear in the Washington meeting referred to above. In this meeting international authorities recommended a variety of treatments including ultraradical mastectomy and partial mastectomy with or without radiation. Two new scientifically controlled current trials comparing the results of radical or modified radical mastectomy with partial mastectomy and removal of nodes were described. So

CHOICES IN
SURGICAL CARE

far in neither of the trials reported were there any differences in survival.

In the past, carefully controlled randomized trials both in this country and abroad have compared the survival of thousands of patients with breast cancer treated by operations varying in extent from *partial mastectomy* (removing the tumor, surrounding tissue, the overlying skin, and the underlying fascia, with reconstruction of the breast) to *ultraradical mastectomy*, in which all the breast, the muscles of the chest wall, and the lymph nodes in the axilla (armpit) are removed (axillary dissection), and in addition the ribs are cut to enable the surgeon to remove the nodes in the chest. (A *simple mastectomy* removes the breast and overlying skin. The nodes in the axilla are not removed.) All sorts of combinations of big operations with or without radiation and little operations with or without radiation have been compared. The results of immediate removal of all nodes have been compared with the results of leaving all nodes in place for at least four months and indefinitely if they do not enlarge. See Note 4 to this chapter for results of ten of these trials. In none of the trials—involving a total of 4,534 patients who have been followed for from five to ten years or more—has the method of treatment made any difference in the proportion of patients surviving.[4] The type of treatment given has, however, made a great deal of difference in the quality of the patient's life, for the radical operations often resulted in swelling of the arm, in pronounced discomfort in the chest wall, and in limitation of motion of the shoulder. Radiation greatly increased the likelihood of these complications. That is why it is so important for you to ask the right questions before submitting to treatment. You should know whether or not the treatment that is proposed is the only effective method. You should know the side effects of the proposed treatment

An Example of Controversy: Diagnosis and Treatment of Cancer of the Breast

and what alternatives there are. Today, with fewer than a third of American surgeons still doing radical mastectomies routinely, none of the proponents of the radical operation can claim that there are no alternatives.

The controversy between those who advise *radical mastectomy*, in which breast muscles and axillary contents are removed, and those who employ the *modified radical mastectomy*, in which the muscles are spared, is being settled rapidly in favor of the smaller and less deforming operation. But there is still controversy as to how to treat a small cancer, the size of a cherrystone or smaller, or one found on x-ray and still so small that it cannot even be felt. There is still disagreement as to whether or not these can be treated successfully by partial mastectomy with reconstruction of the breast, provided that they seem to be localized and that no other deposits of cancer can be found in the biopsy specimen.

The controversy about partial mastectomy is still in its infancy, because until recently in the treatment of cancer very few surgeons ever considered doing any operation less than total mastectomy. Times are changing, however. Careful studies by a number of surgeons and radiotherapists abroad and by a few in this country and Canada have shown that in selected cases when the tumors are small, and when they are localized and not situated near the nipple, wide local excision with or without radiation is as effective as radical operations. For this reason, the National Cancer Institute has authorized Dr. Bernard Fisher and his National Surgical Adjuvant Breast Project, composed of twenty-odd university hospitals and cancer centers, to conduct a randomized trial between modified radical mastectomy and two types of treatment that preserve the breast—i.e., wide local excision with removal of the axillary nodes, and the same operation followed by radiation. If differences in the survival rates of

CHOICES IN
SURGICAL CARE

patients treated by these various methods had already been demonstrated, the National Cancer Institute could not have authorized and funded this trial.

In view of these developments it is more important than ever for women to ask the right questions. If they knew that our government was sponsoring such a trial, many women whose cancers are small, apparently localized, and situated in the periphery of the breast would prefer to have a partial mastectomy with reconstruction of the breast.

There is an even lesser operation sometimes called *lumpectomy*, in which only the tumor is removed. This operation, done to some extent in Europe and more recently in New England, is generally accompanied by radiation. In patients with small, suitably located cancers and with no apparent involvement of nodes, the survival rate has been the same as after radical mastectomy, but the radiation sometimes produces uncomfortable side effects. (See Note 4, item i.)

The list of options in the treatment of cancer of the breast goes on and on. If women knew how to ask the right questions, they would find that in almost any operable cancer of the breast, especially if nodes are not obviously involved, a modified radical mastectomy can be done, removing all the breast and the axillary nodes in such a way that a thick and loose layer of skin and fat is left. A few months later a plastic surgeon can insert a plastic implant to restore the contour of the breast so that any type of evening or bathing dress can be worn without showing deformity or scar. With a bra on, there is nothing to suggest that an operation has been done.

More complicated than a simple restoration of contour but still feasible, if planned in advance, is the *nipple transplant*, in which the original nipple or one fabricated from part of the nipple on the other side or from skin from the labia or thigh is grafted onto the reconstructed breast. At present this

An Example of Controversy:
Diagnosis and Treatment of Cancer of the Breast

operation is not common, because most general surgeons do not know how to do it well. Unless the patient asks specifically for it, there is little incentive for the surgeon to call in a plastic surgeon to help. But all this is changing rapidly, and I believe that in the future, after mastectomy, many of the younger women will want to have their bodily contours restored. All they have to do is to ask for it, because after an operation for almost all operable breast cancers, reconstruction is possible.

Another alternative, suitable mainly for women with small and apparently localized breast cancers, is *subcutaneous* (under-the-skin) *mastectomy*. In this operation the breast tissue and some of the lymph nodes in the armpit are removed, while the skin of the breast and the nipple is left intact. Later a plastic implant is inserted to restore the contour. Often the scar can be so well hidden in the fold of skin under the breast that it is hard to tell which breast was operated on. This operation is not popular with general surgeons but is being done more and more by plastic surgeons who have been better trained in the techniques of preserving the nipple and restoring the contour of the breast.

The surgeons who advocate, or who in selected cases are willing to perform, operations less than radical mastectomy are just as well qualified as those who insist on doing the radical operations. For example, most of the surgeons at Johns Hopkins, where radical mastectomy was first popularized nearly a century ago by Dr. Halsted, now perform the modified radical operation. Within the past five years the surgeons at the Mayo Clinic likewise have switched to the modified radical. In 1974 a survey of breast surgeons in Pennsylvania showed that less than half of the operations for cancer were radical.[5] A similar survey in 1978 would probably show that less than 25 percent were radical. That is why it is such a tragedy when a woman does not know that radical

CHOICES IN SURGICAL CARE

mastectomy is on its way out and as a result accepts the needless discomforts and deformities that the radical operations so often inflict.

The modified radical mastectomy removes all the local cancer and gives as high a chance of cure as any. If one were to pick a single form of treatment for use in all patients with operable breast cancer, the modified radical operation would be the choice. But some women cannot bear the thought of losing the breast. For these women, if their cancers are small, partial mastectomy (with or without radiation) is the best answer. The possibility of having local recurrence or appearance of a new cancer is a little greater than after a modified radical mastectomy, but since the breast is under constant surveillance, any recurrence is apt to be recognized and treated early, before it can jeopardize survival. Partial mastectomy with or without radiation has been used extensively for a number of years in many well-known institutions, including the following, which have repeatedly reported their results in scientific journals:

> University of Toronto (Princess Margaret Hospital)
> Yale University Medical School, New Haven
> Massachusetts General Hospital (Harvard Medical School), Boston
> M. D. Anderson Cancer Center, Houston
> Cleveland Clinic
> Albert Einstein College of Medicine, New York
> Beth Israel Hospital, Boston

In addition, of course, partial mastectomy has been widely used abroad, especially in England, France, and Scandinavia.

There are enormous differences in deformity, discomfort, and disability, depending on what surgeon does the radical

An Example of Controversy:
Diagnosis and Treatment of Cancer of the Breast

operations. In some parts of the country surgeons still use the original Halsted technique of radical mastectomy, cutting paper-thin skin flaps that cling to the bare ribs, or they remove so much skin that to replace it they have to graft skin taken from the thigh. They remove all of the muscles right to the collar bone, so that there is an ugly hollow in the upper chest, making it necessary to wear high-collared dresses to hide the defect. Moreover, the scar is vertical and even goes down the front of the upper arm, where not only is it conspicuous, but it cuts lymphatics that normally drain the fluid from the skin of the arm and thereby increases the patient's chances of having a permanently swollen arm. In other parts of the country surgeons who say they perform radical mastectomies have so modified the original Halsted operation that they leave thick skin flaps, part of the muscle, and use a transverse incision so that the operation is almost indistinguishable from the modified radical mastectomy.

Before consenting to a radical mastectomy, therefore, the knowledgeable patient should spend some time discussing with the surgeon the question of the direction of the incision, the parts of the muscle to be removed, the thickness of the skin flaps, and the use of grafts, all of which decisions have no effect on the chance of cure but exert a strong influence on the time required to heal, on the function of the shoulder, on the likelihood of having a permanently swollen arm, and the comfort and appearance of the chest wall.

The latest contribution to the breast-cancer controversy is from Dr. Oliver Cope, Clinical Professor of Surgery at Harvard and surgeon at the Massachusetts General Hospital. In a recent book entitled *The Breast*,[6] Dr. Cope states flatly that under no circumstance is a mastectomy indicated as the primary treatment of breast cancer. Instead, Dr. Cope recommends local excision of the cancer (the lumpectomy mentioned earlier), followed by radiation given in a specialized

Choices in
Surgical Care

radiation center using a high-powered linear accelerator. If the cancer is advanced, special types of radiation are used without surgery.

Radiologists of another group in Boston, Dr. Martin B. Levene and his associates, recommend the use of "booster" doses of radiation given by implanting wires of radioactive iridium into the area of the tumor. They also radiate the area with a cobalt or linear-accelerator beam. Although their preliminary results are promising and there seem to be few serious side effects or deformities, it is too soon to evaluate the results in terms of long-term control of the cancer.

It is my impression that in properly selected cases these new combinations of minor surgery and radiation may compete effectively with radical surgery.

Since so much depends on what operation or combination of operation and radiation is selected, and upon who is selected to do it, it is important for the patient to inform herself of all possibilities. The treatment advised does not depend at all on the qualifications of the surgeon who advises the treatment. Expert surgeons who are certified by the American Board of Surgery, who are members of honor societies, and who have specialized all their lives in cancer surgery or even in breast surgery may strongly prefer either radical or conservative treatment. So long as the disease is in the same stage and the primary tumor is removed or effectively irradiated, their end results, in terms of survival, are the same regardless of the choice of initial treatment. That is why women should insist on discussing the pros and cons of each type of treatment with their surgeons.

In discussing the choice of operation, women should express their own preferences. Some women to whom the breast is precious may elect to save the breast or to have it reconstructed. Another group of patients, often women with young children, may feel such a sense of responsibility that

An Example of Controversy:
Diagnosis and Treatment of Cancer of the Breast

they are willing to make any sacrifice if they believe it will increase their chance of recurrence-free survival. Another group that often opts for removal of the breast is composed of older women who are no longer sexually active, and want only to be free of worry about local recurrence or appearance of new cancers.

When survival rates appear to be the same regardless of the method of treatment, women should have their choice. It is the duty of the physician to discuss the various options. The table on pp. 22–23 shows the pros and cons of each operation, based upon the recent studies listed in Note 4 (163–165). None of these studies shows a significant difference in survival rates. Since modified radical mastectomy is the operation most commonly used, the results of this operation are considered to be "average" and are used as a yardstick to evaluate the results of other forms of treatment. "Indication" means under what circumstances the treatment is considered to be useful. "Morbidity" means deformity, disability, and discomfort. "Survival" relates to the proportion of patients who, in scientifically controlled trials, have lived for ten years after treatment. Obviously, cancers of comparable size and stage must be compared for these results to be meaningful.

Recent studies continue to question the advantages of radical mastectomy. The most important of the ongoing scientifically controlled and randomized trials is that of the National Surgical Adjuvant Breast Project, which compares the results after radical mastectomy with those after simple mastectomy and also with those after simple mastectomy with irradiation.[7] Now in its seventh year and already involving 1,665 patients from thirty-four institutions in Canada and the United States, this trial is sponsored by the National Cancer Institute under the direction of Dr. Bernard Fisher, Professor of Surgery, University of Pittsburgh Medical School. Pre-

	Indication	Expense	Morbidity	Local Recurrence	Survival	Comment
Ultraradical mastectomy	None	Highest	Very high	Average	Average	Rarely done here or abroad
Radical mastectomy with radiation	None	Very high	Highest	Low	Average or perhaps less than average	Largely abandoned in recent years
Radical mastectomy	None	High	High	Above average	Average	Increasingly replaced by modified version
Modified radical mastectomy	Any patient with invasive cancer	Average	Average	Average	Average	Commonest and most useful operation for invasive cancer
Simple mastectomy with radiation	When cancer in nodes is extensive	Average	Higher than average	Average	Average	Used in England instead of the modified radical
Simple mastectomy with low axillary dissection	Very small cancers or noninvasive cancers	Lower than average	Low	Average	Average	Satisfactory procedure for highly selected favorable cancers
Simple mastectomy with axillary biopsy & implant	Cancers without involvement of nodes	High	Low	Above average*	Average	Somewhat complicated procedure, usually satisfactory but occasionally uncomfortable

	Indication	Expense	Morbidity	Local Recurrence	Survival	Comment
Simple mastectomy with axillary biopsy, implant, & nipple transplant	Cancers without involvement of nodes & not close to nipple	High	Low	Above average*	Average	Most complicated of all reconstructive procedures—surgeon expert in this procedure desirable
Subcutaneous mastectomy with axillary dissection & implant	Noninvasive multicentric or small central cancers	Higher than average	Low	Above average*	Average	Useful in patients who want to save their nipples & are not suitable for partial mastectomy
Local excision (lumpectomy) & radiation	Small, apparently localized cancers	Average	Average	Above average*	Average	Treatment that involves increased morbidity and worry about local recurrence but can be used for almost any small cancer
Partial mastectomy (wide local excision) with or without axillary dissection	Small, apparently localized cancers that are not near the nipple	Lowest	Lowest	Above average*	Average	Not widely performed but successful in all studies in which it has been used—may require later axillary dissection.

For references to the scientifically controlled trials on which this table is based, see Note 4.

*The risk of local recurrence is greater following conservative surgery that does not remove the axillary nodes than following radical surgery that does, but experience has shown that the nodes can be removed if and when the cancer in them becomes palpable and that if they are then removed the chance of survival is just as good as it would have been if the nodes had been removed in the beginning.

CHOICES IN
SURGICAL CARE

liminary results, published in June 1977 in the journal *Cancer*, "fail to demonstrate an advantage for those who had a radical mastectomy."

The most recent publication supporting the concept that radical mastectomy has no advantage over simpler operations with or without radiation is based on the above-mentioned trials and comes from Drs. K. McPherson and M. S. Fox. They write, "The clinical evidence that has accumulated demonstrates persuasively that radical mastectomy offers no greater benefit to the patient than does simple mastectomy. This being the case, what proof is there that limited surgery, such as *tylectomy* [lumpectomy] would not offer an equal benefit to some patients?"[8] They also point out that while "radical mastectomy is no more effective than simple surgery in terms of survival experience and the chances of local or distant recurrence," it costs "more in dollars for surgery and hospital stay and does induce more morbidity, more mutilation, and more traumatic psychological adjustment as well as carrying a greater risk of surgical death."

Radiation—In Which Cases?

In the 1976 Washington meeting, authorities agreed that the routine use of radiation therapy after radical operations was superfluous. One said that rather than prolonging life it actually reduced life expectancy. Another said that in selected cases it was helpful. A third reported superior results by treating the cancer by radiation alone, using a special form of radiation devised by Dr. Pierrequin of Paris, which com-

An Example of Controversy: Diagnosis and Treatment of Cancer of the Breast

bined the conventional variety with radiation from radioactive iridium wires inserted into and around the tumor. Local tumors had been controlled for several years in all of the thirty-odd cases in which the method had been used. What the long-range results would be in terms of the local control of the cancer, the survival of the patient, or the appearance and comfort of the heavily irradiated breast were anyone's guesses.

Clearly, we still know very little about the end results of many of the possible combinations of treatment. One thing, however, is sure. Large randomized trials both here and abroad have shown that radiation after an adequate operation does not increase survival. Since radiation causes complications such as swelling of the arm, skin changes, and stiffness of the shoulder, it should not be used routinely. It should be reserved for special cases, such as a tumor so extensive that all of it cannot be removed or one in the inner quadrant of the breast which sometimes spreads to lymph nodes in the chest. It can be useful also when small cancers have been removed by local excision alone.

Endocrine Therapy— Surgical or Medical?

So far we have been dealing with the primary treatment of breast cancer, about which not even the most knowledgeable authorities agree. Now we come to an even more confusing area but one in which, curiously enough, there is more agreement, even though there is not yet any scientific basis for that

Choices in Surgical Care

agreement. I am referring to manipulating endocrine functions to slow the growth of cancer cells or destroy them.

It has been known for nearly a century that in premenopausal women, removing the ovaries or destroying their function by irradiating them often caused cancers of the breast and their metastases to shrink or disappear. The effect is not permanent, and after a few months or years the cancer begins to grow again. Most physicians have taken the view that since the control is not permanent, there is no use in doing this treatment until a recurrence takes place. They argue that if the ovaries are then removed or irradiated, the cancer will enter a second remission just as long, and the patient will gain just as many months or years of life as she would have if this had been done at the time of the initial treatment. A randomized study in the United States has supported this belief,[9] but two studies abroad suggested that early irradiation of the ovaries in premenopausal women resulted in an increased rate of survival at both five and ten years. In one of these studies, done at the Princess Margaret Hospital in Toronto by Dr. P. J. Fitzpatrick, the premenopausal women whose ovaries were treated by radiation had a significantly increased survival rate ten years later. Similar findings have been observed in experiments with mice, the cure rate being significantly higher in the animals whose ovaries were removed.

Although the question of the effect of removal or irradiation of the ovaries on survival has not been settled for certain, there is an additional consideration which is important for young women who have "favorable" cancers—cancers that probably can be cured. These women, if so treated while still in their thirties, will have only a quarter of the expected risk of getting a new cancer in the other breast, or if a partial mastectomy had been done, in the remnants of the affected breast. The treatment also reduces the amount of normal

An Example of Controversy: Diagnosis and Treatment of Cancer of the Breast

breast tissue, making a new cancer easier to find either by palpation or by x-ray. The trouble is that early menopause brought on by the sudden drop in hormones secreted by the ovary has many side effects and some risks. Small doses of estrogen can counteract these side effects, but no one knows whether this restores the tendency to get breast cancer.

In view of this confused state of our knowledge it is small wonder that physicians do not agree as to the advisability of removing or irradiating the ovaries in premenopausal women. If the decision is left to the woman, she must decide whether she prefers to have menopause induced. If she does this, her breasts will become soft, free from pain, and easier to examine. If she prefers not to interrupt the function of the ovaries, she increases the risk of having a new cancer appear in the other breast, or if a partial mastectomy was done, in the same breast. Certainly, a young woman with a malignant or premalignant tumor of one breast should strongly consider having the ovaries removed or irradiated. In the absence of more definite guidelines, however, the wants, fears, and desires of the patient should be an important part of the decision.

In cases where the cancer has metastasized, even when the cancer and its metastases have responded dramatically and disappeared sooner or later after removal of the ovaries, the cancer starts to grow again. This is because estrogen, the female hormone that stimulates its growth, is formed in the adrenals as well as in the ovaries. The secretion of estrogen can be stopped again by removing the adrenal glands, located over the kidneys, or by removing the pituitary gland, located in the skull at the base of the brain. If the tumor is sensitive to estrogens (for which there are tests), removal of either of these glands gives a good chance that the tumor will shrink again and will not grow again for months or even years. However, both of these operations are major and entail not only discomfort but side effects and risk. To be sure that you will not be subjected to one of these operations unless your cancer has a good chance of being controlled by them, you must insist at the time of your first operation that the tumor tissue be tested for the presence of *estrogen receptors*. If these are present, the tumor probably will shrink when the level of estrogen in the blood is lowered, as it would be by removing the ovaries, adrenals, or pituitary.

Recently a series of drugs known as antiestrogens have been synthesized and a form of treatment called *medical adrenalectomy* has been developed, in which an antihormone, Tamoxifen, and the adrenal hormone, prednisone, are used to neutralize or block the secretion of estrogen. In postmenopausal women with cancers that when tested are shown to have estrogen receptors, and in premenopausal women whose cancers have responded to removal of the ovaries, there is as good a chance of success with medical treatment as with the major operations of removing the adrenal or pituitary glands. It is not yet certain that the remissions induced by medical treatment will last as long as those that follow the operations, but the medical treatment is safe and has few side effects. If a patient has been advised to have the adrenals or pituitary removed, she should inquire also about the medical alternatives.

Chemotherapy—An Open Question

In 1975 Dr. Bonadonna published the results of a randomized trial supported in Italy by our National Cancer Institute in which, when evaluated two years later, patients treated

An Example of Controversy: Diagnosis and Treatment of Cancer of the Breast

for a year after mastectomy by three powerful chemical agents had done spectacularly better than those who had had no chemical treatment. The report was hailed in scientific journals and the press as a breakthrough. Now, a year later, Dr. Bonadonna, a dedicated and objective scientist, reported that in postmenopausal women, chemotherapy had not produced a significant decrease in recurrence or any increase in survival. At the end of three years it was only in women who were still menstruating at the time of the operation that the chemotherapy had been of value.

In most patients the chemotherapy stopped menstruation. This immediately raised the question, Dr. Bonadonna said, as to whether the benefit was due to a direct effect of the chemicals on the tumor or to an indirect effect, by suppressing the activity of the ovaries, pituitary, and adrenals whose hormones stimulate the growth of many breast cancers. If it turns out that the benefits of chemotherapy in premenopausal patients with breast cancer are due to suppression of hormones, it will make it much easier on the patient, because inducing menopause by removal of the ovaries or radiating them is a simpler, less uncomfortable procedure than chemotherapy. Moreover, there are the before-mentioned effective and nontoxic methods of neutralizing estrogen and of controlling its output by the adrenals.

Should women beyond the menopause accept chemotherapy with its side effects of losing hair and of nausea, vomiting, and feeling weak on and off for a year? A year ago it seemed clear that chemotherapy was worthwhile in women whose cancers had involved axillary nodes. Now the whole question is again wide open.

CHOICES IN
SURGICAL CARE

Scans—When Are They Useful?

In recent years there has been a growing tendency for surgeons to order bone and/or liver scans before operating for breast cancer. The scans, done with a radioactive isotope that becomes concentrated in cancer tissue, shows whether or not the cancer has spread to bone or liver. If the cancer has spread to bone, there would be no use performing a mastectomy. Treatment would be by chemicals and/or radiation. When the cancer is large or shows evidence of having spread to lymph nodes scans are clearly indicated, because in these advanced cancers involvement of bone or liver is common. But scans are expensive, and not wholly accurate. Moreover, in patients whose cancers are small and do not seem to have involved the nodes, scans are so rarely positive, and so apt to be wrong, showing a false positive, that few surgeons would advise against removing a potentially curable cancer on the basis of a scan alone. For these reasons many surgeons do not order the expensive scans in patients with small favorable-looking cancers that give no clinical, x-ray, or laboratory evidence of having spread. But if the tumor is large, or if the lymph nodes of the armpit seem to be enlarged on the affected side, the patient should demand a scan before subjecting herself to an unnecessary mastectomy.

An Example of Controversy:
Diagnosis and Treatment of Cancer of the Breast

How to Choose and Who Should Choose

If the world's most knowledgeable medical authorities disagree over the treatment of women's most common type of fatal cancer, we must admit that the patient's guess as to the value of various types of treatments is apt to be just as good as her doctor's. Perhaps the best rule for her to follow is, *in case of doubt, accept the treatment that involves the least deformity, discomfort, disability, and risk of fatal complications.*

Disagreement among physicians occurs for two reasons. First, no good information about end results is yet available. Secondly, there are many areas in which physicians disagree because of traditional beliefs, biases, incentives, or prejudices. The physicians on one side may be as well trained and as competent as those on the other. The patient cannot make a judgment on the basis of the credentials, the integrity, or the personality of her physician. She must insist on knowing the alternatives available to her and the pros and cons of each. Then and only then can she decide which of the proposed treatments she will accept.

The physician should not try routinely to impose his favorite treatment on the patient. Survival depends not on the extent of treatment but rather on whether or not the cancer had already spread before it was removed or destroyed. Since all treatments that destroy or remove the primary cancer and its nearby involved lymph nodes result in the same proportion of long-time survivors, it is clear that the decision as to what treatment will be given must be worked out in a long and frank discussion between the physician and the patient. The day is over when a surgeon can tell a patient, "I know what is best for you; just leave it to me." Today's pa-

CHOICES IN SURGICAL CARE

tient knows enough about breast cancer to want to share in the decisions. There is no reason why she shouldn't do so.

This summary of current medical knowledge and opinions regarding the treatment of breast cancer has been used as a model to indicate how divided medical opinion is even in the treatment of the most common cancer affecting women. In the next two chapters we will see that there are other types of cancer and many other diseases about whose treatment the medical profession is equally divided.

III

Controversy in Other Types of Cancer

Since this book is being written primarily for the benefit of the patient, I am not including controversies about the treatments of rare diseases, but will limit the discussion to those common diseases in which there are striking differences in the risk or in the patient's comfort depending on which form of treatment is chosen. Those that will be discussed represent only about half of the thirty areas of disagreement described in Varco and Delaney's recent surgical test, *Controversy in Surgery*.[1] Many of these controversies involve the treatment of cancer, because the causes and nature of cancer are not yet well understood. Clearly, when there is that much disagreement among surgeons, the patient should try to find out about the alternatives in order to select the treatment that will give the best chance of survival and of living a comfortable life.

CHOICES IN
SURGICAL CARE

Cancer in Situ of the Cervix

Most women are careful to protect themselves against cancer of the cervix (the lower part of the uterus) by having periodic Pap smears. These smears may show varying degrees of abnormal changes up to and including a truly spreading type of cancer. The most important function of a Pap test is to detect precancerous or very early cancerous change, generally referred to as *in-situ cancer* or *cervical intra-epithelial neoplasm*. An in-situ cancer is one that is confined to the most superficial layers of tissue and can be compared to veneer on furniture or to enamel on a refrigerator. It has not invaded the deep tissues. It has no access to blood or lymphatic vessels through which it might spread to distant organs. When the cancer is discovered and destroyed at this stage, all the women who have it are cured; on the other hand, if the cancer is not discovered until it has invaded the cervix and perhaps has spread to the lymph nodes or elsewhere, there is a good chance that in spite of any treatment it will be fatal.

When a Pap smear shows the presence of abnormal cells, tissue specimens must be obtained in order to make a precise diagnosis. After the diagnosis is established there is no agreement on the appropriate treatment of in-situ or noninvasive cancer. Several choices exist, ranging from *hysterectomy* through *conization* (removal of a cone-shaped tissue specimen from the mouth of the uterus) and *cauterization* of very localized lesions on the cervix (located by means of biopsy and microscopic examination) to *cryotherapy* (destruction of the tumor by freezing).

In-situ cancer of the cervix often appears in women who are still in their late teens or early twenties. Many of these women have not yet had babies. If their in-situ cancers are

Controversy in
Other Types of Cancer

treated by hysterectomy there is no hope of pregnancy. If treated by cauterization, conization, or cryosurgery, most women can conceive and deliver normally. For these young women the decision as to whether to have a hysterectomy can have a profound effect on their lives and marriages. Yet, in this common situation gynecologists do not agree about treatment. Some insist on hysterectomy. Others are content to cone out the cervix.

A young woman who wants to have children in the future should know that there are alternatives to hysterectomy. In any case, if the entire uterus is not removed it is important that Pap tests be carried out at regular intervals in order to monitor the effectiveness of treatment. The following table summarizes the advantages and disadvantages of hysterectomy compared with lesser procedures.

	Cost	Dis-com-fort	Risk	Side Effects	Possible Complications	Survival
Cryosurgery	+	0	0	0	Discharge (temporary)	Same*
Cauterization or Conization	+	0	0+	0	Bleeding	Same*
Hysterectomy	+++	++	++	Sterility	Intestinal obstruction; embolism; severing of ureter	Same

*Conization or cryosurgery cures most cancers in situ, but not all. In a few cases the Pap smear remains positive and it is necessary to repeat the conization or remove the whole uterus. The ultimate cure rate, however, is the same.

The advantages of conization over hysterectomy mainly concern the patients who are young and may want to have children. When cancer in situ of the cervix is found in a woman who has already had all the children she wants, the

Choices in Surgical Care

situation is quite different. There are some definite advantages to hysterectomy.

Women who have had hysterectomies need have no further worries about contraception or abortion. They do not have to take the contraceptive pill, which carries with it a slightly increased risk of fatal blood-clotting disorders, and has various side effects such as vaginitis and breast discomfort. Besides this, the hysterectomy, with removal of ovaries too, gives complete protection against death from three fairly common types of cancer—those of cervix, endometrium, and ovary. In addition, as we pointed out before, women who have their ovaries removed while they are still in their thirties reduce their chance of contracting cancer of the breast to only a quarter of the normal expectancy. Since one woman in fifteen contracts breast cancer at some time in her life, and since at least half of those who do will die of it, this means that removing the ovaries has saved three-quarters of these (i.e., one woman in forty, or approximately 2.5 percent of the women treated) from dying of breast cancer. One must also consider the remote possibility of fatal complications from pregnancy or abortion. Taking all these factors into consideration, and remembering, too, that in healthy young women the mortality rate of elective hysterectomy (i.e., the risk of dying from complications of the operation) is only about one in a thousand, it is clear that it is safer to have a hysterectomy than not to. This is probably why about half of all doctors' wives have had the operation, a higher percentage than in the population at large. It is hard, therefore, to accuse doctors of advising too many hysterectomies or to imply that they perform so many of them solely because of financial considerations.

We know that menopause, including early menopause brought about by removal of the ovaries, causes many changes in the body. These include unpleasant hot flashes,

Controversy in Other Types of Cancer

tensions, dryness of the vagina, and in the long run some weakening of the bones due to loss of calcium and perhaps an increase in the pace of hardening of the arteries, causing heart disease or stroke. In women who have had their ovaries removed, all of these effects can be prevented by giving continuous low-dose treatment with estrogen pills. But the question is, does estrogen, so given, neutralize the effects that removal of the ovaries has given in preventing cancer of the breast? Incredible as it may seem, no study has ever been done that either affirms or denies the possibility. We simply don't know. My guess is that if minimal doses of estrogen are given continuously (instead of the twenty-one-day cycles of doses given when the uterus is left in), removal of the ovaries would continue to give significant protection against cancer of the breast.

Cancer of the Head and Neck

There are too many different kinds of cancer of the head and neck, and too many different combinations of surgery and/or radiation treatment, to make it possible to discuss treatment in detail. Suffice it to say that good radiation therapy can supplement radical operations, or if the cancer is extensive, radiation can be used instead of radical operations, for palliation. The area of controversy worth discussing is the type of operation done on the neck to remove lymph nodes to which the cancers may have metastasized but in which no cancer can be felt at the time.

The standard technique of radical neck dissection was first described in the latter part of last century by my father, Dr.

CHOICES IN SURGICAL CARE

George Crile, Sr. At that time cancers of the mouth, tongue, face, and lip were usually huge by the time they were diagnosed, and had metastasized extensively to the lymph nodes of the neck. When head cancers involve nodes, they soon invade the node's capsule, break through, and invade surrounding tissues. For this reason radical neck dissection removes the surrounding tissues, including important muscles and nerves.

	Cost	Discomfort	Risk	Side Effects	Possible Complications	Survival
Radical neck	+ ++	+ ++	+	+ ++ (cosmetic)	++	++
Modified radical neck	+ ++	++	0+	0	+	++*

*Cure rate is same in properly selected cases that are not advanced.

Today, the situation in cancer of the head and neck is quite different. The cancers tend to be small. In most cases no metastasis in nodes can be felt. Large metastases that have invaded the capsule are rare. In all other cases just as effective a dissection can be done without damage to nerve or muscle and without producing significant deformity or disability. The incision can be the same as the radical operation, the exposure of underlying tissue is the same, the same number of nodes can be removed—and all of this can be done without mutilation. Many head-and-neck surgeons are using such modifications of the radical dissection, but some still persist in performing the standard operation. If no nodes or only small ones are palpable and if a radical neck dissection is suggested, it is important to ask about alternatives.

Controversy in
Other Types of Cancer

Cancer of the Larynx

In heavy smokers, and especially in men, cancer of the larynx is common. There are two types. The first, and the most common, is the type that involves the vocal cords. Fortunately this type causes hoarseness early so that most patients recognize that something is wrong and consult a doctor in time. The other types of laryngeal cancer do not affect the vocal cords. These are much more dangerous because they cause no symptoms until they are advanced and give pain or give rise to metastasis in the lymph nodes of the neck, by which time most of them are incurable.

The earliest type of cancer that involves the vocal cords is cancer in situ which has not yet invaded the underlying tissues. In most cases this can be cured by one or more "strippings" of the vocal cord in which the cancer-bearing lining of the larynx is stripped away. The lining soon regenerates and leaves the vocal cords and the voice quite normal.

The next degree of malignancy is the early invasive cancer. This is a true cancer with malignant potential, but when it is small, superficial, and does not seem to have metastasized it can be cured just as effectively by radiation as by surgery, provided of course that the radiation is given by a specialist with good equipment in a recognized center.

If the cancer of the vocal cord is larger and more invasive than the minimum lesion described above, but is still limited to one cord, it can be treated by partial laryngectomy, with removal of the cord on the affected side only. In cases in which this results in an extremely hoarse or "breathy" voice, a reconstructive procedure can inject a plastic into the larynx to narrow the opening and improve the voice. But this remains one of the controversial areas of laryngeal surgery, because many surgeons prefer to operate and many radio-

Choices in Surgical Care

therapists prefer to treat the cancer first by radiation. They advise removing the cord or larynx only in those cases in which the radiation fails to control the cancer.

When the tumor is large and invasive or when nodes are involved, there is general agreement that total laryngectomy and radiation combined offer the best chances of control. Total removal of the larynx is an unpleasant operation that involves a permanent opening through which the patient breathes. The only way he can speak is by using an artificial "voice box" or by learning to swallow air and to belch it out through the esophagus into the mouth, a feat that with training is accomplished successfully by many patients.

	Cost	Discomfort	Risk	Side Effects	Possible Complications	Survival
Total laryngectomy	++ ++	+ ++	++	++ ++ Loss of voice	++	+ ++
Partial laryngectomy	+ ++	++	+	++ Hoarseness	+	+ ++ (in selected cases)
Radiation	+ ++	+	+	+	+	+ ++ (in selected cases)

Unfortunately this operation of total laryngectomy is the one most commonly recommended for another type of laryngeal cancer, the type that does not involve the vocal cords but the tissues above them. Sometimes in the cancers of the upper part of the larynx it is possible to do a partial

Controversy in Other Types of Cancer

laryngectomy, removing the cancer-bearing tissue but sparing the vocal cords. In such cases the voice remains normal. But again in such cases radiotherapists often urge a trial of radiation therapy and advise operation only in those cases in which treatment fails. The same recommendations are made by some radiotherapists in those cases where the cancer is so extensive that to cure it by operation all of the larynx would have to be removed.

Radiation is not without its discomforts and side effects, the most serious of which is the rare but important complication of *chondritis,* which destroys the cartilage of the larynx. This can result in infection, discomfort, and deformity.

From the above description of the treatments available for laryngeal cancer it must be clear that there is no firm agreement among surgical and radiological specialists. The best results are obtained and the best opinions are rendered when members of the two specialties consult and work together. Although not all surgeons would agree, it is my feeling that in cases in which the patient is threatened with severe hoarseness or loss of voice from the recommended operation he should inquire into the possibility of trying radiation first and resorting to radical surgery only if a few months later there is still evidence of an active tumor.

Cancer of the Lung

Cancer of the lung is one of the commonest and most dangerous kinds of cancer. Fewer than 5 percent of the patients are cured by any or all methods of treatment.

In the 1930s, when the technique of chest surgery was

Choices in Surgical Care

being developed and when good anesthesia for open-chest surgery first became available, surgeons began for the first time to operate on patients with cancer of the lung. Radical operations were done, in which all of one lung was removed along with as many of the nearby lymph nodes as possible. However, one distinguished chest surgeon contended that removal of the entire lung was both dangerous and unnecessary. He maintained that in most cases better results in terms of survival could be obtained by removing only the affected lobe of one lung. *Lobectomy* this was called, and at the time it was considered by most surgeons to be a totally inadequate treatment of cancer.

Finally, after bitter debates and as a result of the cooperation of a number of surgeons, a clinical trial was planned in which one group of surgeons would remove all the lung and Dr. Richard Overholt and his group would do mainly lobectomies. Time passed, and it was found that, just as Overholt had predicted, more patients were alive five years after lobectomy than after removal of the entire lung. This was not because the cancer was more effectively cured by the lesser operation, but because many of the patients who had the entire lung removed died because they didn't have enough lung tissue left. They were smokers, and in addition to their cancers they had such severe emphysema that they could not survive the loss of the lung. This is a historic example of an operation that seemed clearly to be the best operation for the eradication of cancer but which was not the best operation for the survival of the patient.

Fortunately, as a result of the controlled studies and careful reports that were done twenty years ago, there is now a general agreement about how cancers of the lung should be treated. The large central ones still require removal of the lung. The small peripheral ones can be treated more safely and just as effectively by lobectomy or even by resection of

Controversy in Other Types of Cancer

a segment of the lung. The trouble is that usually, by the time the cancer is diagnosed, it already has spread through the system.[2] For that reason what is done locally makes little difference. The main lesson to be learned about cancer of the lung is to stop smoking cigarettes.

Melanomas

Controversy still rages over the treatment of melanomas, the black skin tumors that arise in moles. These highly malignant cancers spread both to lymph nodes and throughout the system. The probability of distant metastasis depends chiefly on the size of the tumor and on the depth to which it invades the tissues.

All surgeons agree that the melanoma should be excised widely, some advocating taking also the underlying tissue, including the fascia that covers the muscle. One well-qualified scientist, however, has produced statistics to prove that there is *more* metastasis when the fascia is removed. Some surgeons take so much skin that a graft must be used to cover the defect, whereas others leave enough skin so that the defect can be closed. These details make little difference if the melanoma is not in a conspicuous area like the face; healing is the same in any event.

What does make a difference is the way the regional lymph nodes are treated. In the case of a melanoma of the leg, for example, the lymph nodes in the groin would come into question.

Some surgeons believe that if the nodes are not palpably involved, it is not necessary to do a radical dissection of the

CHOICES IN
SURGICAL CARE

groin. The nodes can be observed closely, and if anything is felt, they then can be removed. Some authorities, including Dr. Neville Davis of Australia, who has written extensively on the subject, see no reason to remove the nodes if they are not palpably involved. Some have proposed that to remove the nodes is inviting disaster, because to do so blocks the flow of lymph and traps cancer cells in the lymphatic vessels. These cells, which otherwise would have been swept to the lymph nodes and mostly destroyed there by lymphocytes, may grow in the lymph spaces of the skin and give rise to many new cancers between the original tumor and the nodes.

Another large group of surgeons believe that there is grave danger in leaving in the nodes. Cancer, they say, will be apt to grow in the nodes and spread elsewhere in the body before it can be recognized and removed. The arguments are the same that have gone on for years about removing the nodes of the armpit in patients with breast cancer.

This was the situation in respect to the treatment of melanoma until September 1977, when the *New England Journal of Medicine* published the results of a study sponsored by the World Health Organization and involving seventeen cancer centers.[3] Five hundred and fifty-three patients with melanomas of arms or legs and with no apparent involvement of the regional lymph nodes were put at random into one of two groups. The patients in the first group were treated by both wide excision of the melanoma and radical dissection of the regional lymph nodes. Those of the second group were treated by wide excision only. Later, if tumor appeared in the nodes, as it did in 24 percent of the cases, the nodes were dissected. If tumor did not appear, no further operation was done. At the end of five years and also at eight years, there was no difference in the proportion of patients surviving. Thus, at no increased risk, 76 percent of the patients who were

[44]

Controversy in Other Types of Cancer

treated by wide excision only were able to avoid the danger and deformity of radical node dissection. In the words of the authors, "Elective lymph node dissection in malignant melanoma of the limbs does not improve the prognosis and is not recommended when patients can be followed at intervals of three months."

Thus, by a single concerted international effort, an age-old controversy has been settled in favor of the comfort and well-being of the patient. When the involvement of the nodes becomes apparent only after the original tumor has been removed, 30 percent of the patients still are cured by node dissection.

	Cost	Dis-com-fort	Risk	Side Effects	Possible Complications	Survival
Immediate Node Dissection	+ ++	++	0+	++ ++	+ ++	Same
No Dissection or	+	+	0	+	+	Same
Delayed Node Dissection	+ ++	++	0+	++ ++	+ ++	

In all cases it is assumed that the nodes are not palpably involved at the time of the initial operation.

From the above study it is clear that it makes little or no difference whether or not the surgeon removes nodes that do not seem to be involved. But in other ways it does make a great deal of difference to the patient. If the melanoma is on the arm and the nodes in the armpit are removed, the arm may become permanently swollen, unsightly, and uncomfortable. This complication of massive swelling of the limb is even more apt to occur and can be even more crippling when a radical dissection of the groin is done for a melanoma of the leg.

Cancer of the Pancreas

I had just started to practice surgery when Dr. Allen Whipple reported the first case of pancreatic cancer treated by radical resection of part of the pancreas, the lower part of the stomach, and the duodenum. Intrigued by this brave leap forward, I entered the field and promptly performed the seventh successful *pancreaticoduodenectomy* to be reported. My enthusiasm for the operation remained unabated for nearly twenty years. I was an incorrigible optimist, and felt sure that sooner or later I would do the radical operation on a patient with a cancer of the pancreas and cure him. But finally I gave up. None of my patients with cancer of the pancreas nor those of my colleagues at the Cleveland Clinic had survived for five years. I went back to the treatment that had been in use before Whipple devised the radical operation.

Cancer of the head of the pancreas blocks the flow of bile from the liver to the intestine and causes jaundice. The operation used before the Whipple operation merely bypassed the blockage by connecting the gallbladder to the intestine. No attempt was made to treat the cancer. The jaundice cleared, the patient felt better. Although eventually the patient was bound to die of cancer, he might live in comfort for months or even years before succumbing. My patients lived longer on an average after bypass than after the radical operations, mainly because so many patients died as a direct result of the latter.

Controversy in Other Types of Cancer

The radical operation for cancer of the pancreas is the biggest, longest, most intricate, and most dangerous operation in general surgery. It takes some surgeons as long as twelve hours to do, although a few can complete it in three hours. Its mortality rate (the incidence of death as a direct result of complications of the operation) depends on the skill and experience of the surgeon, the reported rates varying from 7 percent to more than 50 percent. The average mortality rate reported by the Hospital Audit System is 32 percent.

High mortality rates might be justified if an operation effected a high proportion of cures, but, unfortunately, only 1 percent of the patients operated on for cancer of the pancreas live five years with no recurrence. To have a third of the patients die right away as a result of an operation that will cure one patient in a hundred does not make sense. In my opinion, more patients would live more months in more comfort if surgeons would do only a bypass instead of trying to cure cancer of the pancreas by radical operations. An exception might be made in the rare case of a relatively young person with a very small and apparently localized cancer, or in the case of a physician who has specialized and has a very low mortality rate. A comparison of the two operations is as follows:

	Cost	Discomfort	Risk	Side Effects	Possible Complications	Survival
Radical pancreaticoduodenectomy	++ ++	++ ++	++ ++ ++	++ + ++	++ + ++	0+ (less than 1%)
Bypass	++	++	++	0	+	0

CHOICES IN
SURGICAL CARE

Cancer of the Prostate Gland

(See also Prostate Gland—Benign Enlargement
in Chapter IV.)

Cancer of the prostate is by far the commonest cancer in older men. If the prostate glands of men beyond the age of fifty who have died of causes other than disease of the prostate are examined carefully, 35 percent of them are found to contain microscopic areas of noninvasive cancer similar to those that are found in cancer in situ of the cervix. Most of these do not go on to become true invasive cancers, but nevertheless enough of them do progress to make cancer of the prostate the most common cause of death from cancer in older men.

Most older men are well aware of the danger of cancer and view the prostate gland with deep concern. What can they do to prevent the development of cancer of the prostate? The answer is, "Almost nothing."

The reason that so little can be done about treating cancer of the prostate by surgery or radiation is that it does not kill by local extension but by a strong tendency to spread and metastasize through the blood to all parts of the body, especially to bone. As often as not, it is the pain from a metastasis in the bone, rather than any local symptom or sign, that first calls the patient's attention to the existence of prostatic cancer. Even if the cancer does show itself first by blocking urination instead of by symptoms of metastasis, usually by that time it has spread elsewhere. That is why radical operations on the prostate, or even radical irradiation of the prostate, usually control the local disease, but may not prevent the distant spread. Fortunately, however, in nearly half the cases the distant

Controversy in Other Types of Cancer

spread is controlled for varying periods of time and sometimes permanently arrested by endocrine treatment. This is done either by removing the cells in the testicles that make the male hormone (testosterone) or by feeding the female hormone, estrogen (usually in the form of stilbestrol), or by a combination of both.

When a patient with symptoms of prostatic disease is first seen, a rectal examination is done to determine the size of the prostate and what it feels like. Cancers are very hard and some of them may be so fixed to surrounding tissues that the urologist can be quite sure that malignancy is present. To confirm this diagnosis a needle biopsy can be done. After proving that the tumor is malignant, there are three quite different methods of treatment, each of which is espoused by a number of well-trained, skillful, and respected urologists who argue among themselves incessantly as to which is best. Some urologists use all of the treatments, selecting the one that they think is appropriate for the individual case.

1. Radical prostatectomy. In the 1950s, when hopes for radical surgery were at their peak, *radical prostatectomy* was in vogue. This involved a very destructive operation, which removed the prostate and surrounding tissues and lymph nodes and left the patient not only impotent but also sometimes incontinent, with no control over urination. The operation has not been proven to cure any more cancers than does endocrine treatment. Yet, in spite of its side effects, it still is sometimes done in special cases. Unfortunately, there are some urologists who make special cases out of ordinary cases and who do the radical operation more often than most of their colleagues think necessary. That is why the patient should always inquire about alternatives. Not only

CHOICES IN SURGICAL CARE

is the immediate risk of the radical operation much higher, in terms of the chance of dying as a direct result of the operation, but the discomforts and disabilities are much greater.

2. Transurethral resection. When the prostate is blocking urination, an illuminated instrument is inserted through the penis, and under direct vision the surgeon cuts out the part of the prostate gland that is blocking the urethra. Following this, either the patient is given estrogen, or the part of the testicle that makes the male sex hormone is removed, or both. Estrogen causes temporary impotence for as long as it is taken. Removal of the bulk of the testicle also may reduce potency, but when estrogen is stopped or when the male hormone is given, potency (and also the cancer) usually return. This method of treatment involves little discomfort, few side effects other than impotence, and minimal expense.

3. Radiation therapy. There is good evidence that radiation therapy is just as effective as surgery in controlling the local cancer,[4] but radiation can have side effects such as irritation of the bladder with uncontrollable urgency of urination, and sometimes it also causes a very uncomfortable irritation of the rectum. Occasionally, as a rare side effect, there can be permanent damage to bladder or rectum. In about 25 percent of the cases there is impotence. To prevent these complications of high doses of radiation given to the pelvic area, radon seeds are sometimes implanted into the prostate to give a high dose of radiation to this area without significant

Controversy in Other Types of Cancer

damage to surrounding structures. Radiation costs about as much as transurethral resection but takes two months instead of less than a week.

In patients who have microscopic cancer of the prostate that is discovered accidentally in the course of examining the tissues removed at the time of treatment of a benign enlargement of the prostate, some urologists advise no treatment at all. They are aware that 50 percent of men over seventy have such microscopic areas of cancer in their prostates, and they know that the vast majority of these do not become invasive and never cause any trouble. It is time enough to worry about the cancer when it begins to give symptoms. This is because if the cancer is of the undifferentiated, rapidly growing type, it will have spread to distant organs before its presence could have been detected, whereas the slowly growing, differentiated type that is by far the most common may never give symptoms or metastasize and usually can be controlled by endocrine treatment. The same philosophy of treatment applies also to small cancers of the prostate that seem to be localized and which give no symptoms except those of obstructing the flow of urine. Many of these, especially in older men, can be treated by transurethral resection alone. This relieves the symptoms and the patient is apt to die of other causes before the slowly growing tumor recurs. Moreover, there is little, if any, tendency for the differentiated, slow-growing type to change into the more aggressive variety.

The following table compares the various treatments for cancer of the prostate. Before accepting one or another, you should evaluate all of the alternatives and choices.

CHOICES IN SURGICAL CARE

	Cost	Dis-com-fort	Risk	Side Effects	Possible Complications	Survival
Trans-urethral resection & endocrine therapy	+++	++	+	+[A]	+	Same
Radiation	+++	++[B]	0	++	++	Same
Radical prostatec-tomy	++++	+++	+++	+ ++[C]	+++	Same

*There has been no adequately controlled study to prove that survival is the same regardless of treatment, but the lack of agreement among conservative surgeons, radical surgeons, and radiotherapists suggests that the differences, if any, are small. This is because the rapidly growing cancers usually have spread to distant organs before they can be recognized and because the slowly growing ones respond so well to treatment with estrogen.

[A]All patients are impotent as long as estrogen is taken.
[B]Much discomfort early due to irritation, but this usually subsides.
[C]Much depends on the skill of the surgeon. In the hands of experts only 5 percent have incontinence of urine.

Small, Low-lying Cancers of the Rectum

If a cancer is high in the rectum or above the rectum, in the lowest part of the large bowel, it can be removed by what is known as an *anterior resection*. The tumor-bearing segment of bowel is removed and the cut end of the colon is sewn to the cut end of the rectum so that continuity is restored and the bowels move normally.

Controversy in Other Types of Cancer

If the cancer is located so low in the rectum that it cannot be removed completely without sacrificing the lower part of the rectum, it is impossible to join the ends of the bowel together and restore continuity. The commonest form of treatment of such a cancer, but not necessarily either the safest or the most acceptable, is the radical removal of all of the rectum and the surrounding lymph nodes. This procedure is known as an *abdominoperineal resection*. It necessitates a permanent opening on the abdominal wall, a *colostomy*, through which the bowels are emptied for the rest of the patient's life. But there are alternatives.

The first and most radical of the alternatives is the *pull-thru* operation, which can be used for many low-lying cancers, and has the advantage of not necessitating a colostomy. In the pull-thru operation the lower rectum is removed and the cut end of the colon is pulled down and through the muscles that control the anus. Later the excess bowel is trimmed off and the cut end attached to the skin. This operation is not widely done by unspecialized general surgeons. To obtain the best results and to retain continence requires the services of a surgeon with a special interest in this field. The pull-thru operation cannot be done in all cases, because the tumor may be too low or may be invading too deeply. Moreover, after this operation, although the bowels are emptied in the ordinary anal position instead of through a colostomy on the abdomen, often there is less than satisfactory control.

The second alternative is treatment by *nonpenetrating radiation* provided from a special, high-powered machine and given through a special tube, inserted into the rectum. The treatment involves very little discomfort and is given without anesthesia and without hospitalization. It

Choices in Surgical Care

has practically no complications. Sometimes two or three treatments are required before the tumor is destroyed completely. In the rare cases in which the tumor is not controlled, an operation can still be done. This method of treatment was devised by radiotherapist Jean Papillon of Lyons, France, and has been used by himself and others for more than ten years with signal success. Its limitations, as we will see later, is that it takes no account of the metastases of the cancer that might be in the lymph nodes and it cannot be used in large tumors that encircle the bowel.

The final alternative is *electrocoagulation*, which, like radiation therapy, involves local destruction of the tumor, in this case by burning it out. It can be used only in small or medium-sized cancers of the rectum. The operation is done under light anesthesia or regional block (an injection similar to the novocaine given by the dentist). It involves little or no hospitalization or discomfort. Its disadvantage, like that of local radiation, is that potentially involved nodes are not removed.

Let us examine the statistics and see if it is really important to remove the regional lymph nodes as in the much more radical operations of pull-thru or the abdominoperineal resection. Both of the radical operations carry a variable but always significant mortality rate—i.e., a chance that the patient will die, not later as a result of the disease, but quickly as a result of the operation. Electrocoagulation, on the other hand, involves no significant risk, and local radiation can be given with no risk at all. In contrast to the low risk of the two types of local treatment, it has been reported that in the Veterans Administration Hospitals, which probably have mortality rates that are average for the country, the mortality rate for the radical abdominoperineal resection is 10 percent. In at least one university hospital it has been reported

Controversy in
Other Types of Cancer

to be as high as 18 percent. If rates like this are reported, one can be sure that even higher ones exist, but have not been mentioned in the surgical literature. The lowest mortality rate ever reported in a large series was 1.8 percent from St. Mark's Hospital, London. Thus, there is a tenfold disparity between the lowest mortality rate and the highest: It makes a big difference who does the operation.

When deciding whether to have a low-lying, small to medium-sized cancer of the rectum treated by the radical operation or by electrocoagulation, the mortality rate of the big operation (as done by the individual surgeon) must be weighed against the nearly nil mortality of the other methods of treatment. The relative merits of the two methods, therefore, depend largely on the mortality rate that the radical operation has in the hands of the surgeon who does it. Consider these figures:

Of 100 patients with small, low rectal cancers,

- 70 patients have no metastasis in nodes and therefore derive no advantage from the radical operation as opposed to radiation or electrocoagulation.

- 30 patients have metastasis in nodes. But by the time cancers have spread to nodes, 80 percent of them are incurable. Hence, 24 of these 30 will die of their cancers even if radical operations are done and the involved nodes are removed. Only 6 will be cured.

What price is paid to save the lives of these six patients with involved nodes? Since the average mortality rate of the radical operation is 10 percent, ten of the hundred patients

Choices in Surgical Care

would have died as a result of the operation in order to save six from dying of cancer. That is why it is important for the patient to know not only what the average risk of the operation is, but also what the risk is at the hospital in which the operation will be done and in the hands of the surgeon who will do it.

In addition to the risk, the discomfort, expense, and the permanent colostomy resulting from the radical operation must be weighed in the decision. After the lesser treatments, the bowels move in the normal way.

A further factor must also be considered. Most patients with rectal cancer are in their sixties and have a normal life expectancy of only about ten years. If they die as a result of a radical operation they die right away, whereas if they die as a result of cancer left in nodes they usually live comfortably for between five and ten years, thus living out half of their normal life expectancy. One can easily calculate that in terms of saving months or years of comfortable life, the radical operation must be done with a mortality rate of 3 percent or less before it can compete with the lesser treatments. There are very few general hospitals whose mortality rates approach this figure. That is why, in order for you to be able to make up your mind as to which type of treatment you will accept, the hospital should be required to furnish you with that hospital's mortality rates for standard operations. Without this information it will be difficult to decide both where to have your operation done and which treatment to accept.

Electrocoagulation treatment for rectal cancer has been known for years. As far back as 1940, Dr. Abraham Strauss in Chicago was reporting excellent results following burning out of the cancer by electrocoagulation. Dr. W. F. Wassink in the Netherlands had done the same, and so had the surgeons at the Mayo Clinic. In selected cases, Dr. John Madden of New York and also surgeons at the Cleveland Clinic have

Controversy in Other Types of Cancer

reported better results following electrocoagulation than after radical operations in similar cases; yet the operation has not gained widespread popularity among surgeons.[5]

Not all cases are suitable for electrocoagulation. If the tumor is too large, destroying it causes stricture of the rectum. If it invades too deeply, it may be difficult or impossible to cure by electrocoagulation or superficial radiation therapy. But experience has shown that even in cases when electrocoagulation fails to destroy all of the cancer, the radical operation can still be done and with results, in terms of cure, as satisfactory as if it had been done in the first place. That is why it is quite incomprehensible why this method of treatment is so seldom used.

It would be easy to say that coagulation is not used extensively because radical operations command fees of $1,000 or more, whereas insurance companies pay only $100 or $200 for the lesser treatments. This may play a part, but it does not tell the whole story. Even in the socialized countries the radical resection remains popular. I can explain this paradox only on the basis of the characteristics of the surgeon's personality, or perhaps on his lack of personal knowledge of the good results that can be obtained by coagulation or radiotherapy.

A surgeon likes to operate and enjoys the technical aspects of surgery. If he didn't enjoy them he would not have taken the years of training required to become certified in this specialty. During the years of training there are certain operations that, because of their size, danger, and drama, are exceptionally challenging to the young surgeon. High among these is the abdominoperineal resection. Then, too, this operation, removing in one vast block the cancer and the bowel and all the tissue and lymph nodes around it, seems to embody what twenty years ago was called "the principle of sound cancer surgery by *en bloc* dissection."

CHOICES IN
SURGICAL CARE

But what of the risk of the operation, of the operative mortality? Most surgeons are optimists, and many of them tend to remember their successes and to forget their failures. Most, if they have not investigated their own mortality rates and are asked to guess them, underestimate them by 50 percent. At least that is what I found when I checked on myself. I believe, therefore, that surgeons who do the radical operation routinely are sincere in their belief that they are giving the best possible treatment. That is why it should be the responsibility of the hospital to know the mortality rate of each operation and to see to it that those surgeons who have too high a proportion of postoperative deaths are not allowed to do the big and dangerous operations.

The following is a comparison of the various treatments for small, low-lying cancers of the rectum. In addition, radiation may be given before the operation or chemotherapy may be given afterward. The former may be of value but there is no proof. To date, chemotherapy has not appeared to increase survival.

	Cost	Dis-com-fort	Risk	Side Effects	Possible Complications	Survival
Abdomino-perineal	++ ++	++ ++	++ ++	++ ++ Colostomy	++ ++	See Note 1
Pull-thru	++ ++	+ ++	++ ++	++ Incontinence	++ ++	See Note 1
Electro-coagulation*	+	0	0+	0	Occasional Bleeding	See Note 2
Radiation*	+	0	0	0	0	See Note 2

1. Depends on mortality rate of individual surgeon.
2. Equal to radical operation if average mortality of radical operation is counted.

*Applicable for cure only in small or medium-sized cancers.

Controversy in
Other Types of Cancer

Cancers of the Skin

Cancers of the skin are common in white people who have been exposed to the sun, ultraviolet light, or radiation. When cancers occur on the skin of the body or extremities it usually is easy to cut them out and close the wound. But when they are large and occur on the face or lips there is often not enough tissue to close the defect without deformity or the use of a conspicuous skin graft. In such cases, nonsurgical methods of treatment should be investigated.

Until recently *surgery* and *radiation* were the only accepted methods of treating cancer of the skin. In cancer of the lip, radiation cured about as many patients as surgery did, and the deformity was less. Recently other methods of treating skin cancer have been developed. In terms of cure the results in selected cases are equal to those of surgery. In terms of the cosmetic result, they are vastly superior. I am speaking of the local use of *chemicals, electrosurgery* (burning), and *cryotherapy* (freezing). These are of especial value in the scaly premalignant keratoses and in wide, superficial, basal-cell cancers that do not tend to invade the underlying tissues.

These new methods of treatment are used primarily by dermatologists, not by surgeons. That is why if a surgeon advises wide excision of a cancer of the face with or without skin graft, it would be worthwhile asking for a second opinion from a dermatologist. The box score is as follows:

CHOICES IN SURGICAL CARE

	Cost	Dis-com-fort	Risk	Side Effects	Possible Complications	Survival
Surgery with or without graft	++	++	+	+ ++ Scar	+	++ ++
Radiation	++	+	0	+ Scar	0+	++ ++
Chemical treatment	++	+	0	+ Scar	0	++ ++*
Electrosurgery and cryotherapy	+	+	0	+ Scar	0	++ ++*

*Except in invading cancers.

Cancer of the Thyroid

The commonest kind of cancer of the thyroid is the *papillary cancer* (*papillary* means shaped like a papilla or nipple). It is common in children and in young women who in the past have had radiation treatment to the neck for enlargement of the thymus, lymph nodes, tonsils, adenoids, or for eczema or acne. For the past thirty years the treatment of this kind of cancer has been bitterly controversial. The argument has been chiefly between surgeons who were more or less specialized in surgery of the thyroid, and those who had specialized in treating cancers of the mouth, throat, and neck, so-called "head-and-neck surgeons."

The surgeons who had long been acquainted with the thyroid knew that in people under the age of forty, papillary

Controversy in Other Types of Cancer

cancers were almost benign in their behavior, rarely spread to distant organs, and that even though the lymph nodes in the neck were often extensively involved, simple removal of these nodes usually effected a complete cure. They knew also that most of the papillary cancers in young people would stop growing and often regress or even disappear when the patient was given enough thyroid medicine by mouth to suppress the output of the pituitary's thyroid-stimulating hormone. For these reasons, and mainly because with conservative treatment they knew that their patients would have normal life expectancies, these surgeons treated their patients by operations which simply removed most of the thyroid and the affected nodes, and they did this without leaving ugly scars or deformities.

Many of the head-and-neck surgeons viewed papillary cancer of the thyroid in a totally different light, insisting that it was a dangerous disease that must be attacked by radical removal of all of the thyroid, the main muscles of the neck, sacrificing the nerve that goes to the shoulder, and removing the jugular vein. This involved a conspicuous vertical incision, a striking deformity of the neck, a shoulder droop leading to troublesome arthritis, and a significant, immediate mortality from complications of the operation. At the same time, total removal of the thyroid involved a significant incidence of tetany, a permanent lowering of blood calcium, resulting from accidental removal of the tiny parathyroid glands, which control the level of calcium in the blood. If the tetany is not controlled by taking appropriate medicine, severe muscle cramps and often cataracts ensue.

CHOICES IN SURGICAL CARE

	Cost	Dis-com-fort	Risk	Side Effects	Possible Complications	Survival
Radical neck dissection	+ ++	+ ++	+	+ ++	++	++ ++
Modified radical neck	++	+	0+	0	+	++ ++

From 1940 through 1975—a period of nearly thirty-five years—the pros and cons of these two methods of treatment were debated heatedly on the podium and in print. Finally, the most prominent supporters of the radical operation capitulated and began to modify their radical operations to produce satisfactory cosmetic and functional results. But some surgeons still persist in doing radical surgery for this least dangerous of all metastasizing cancers. All of them are well aware of the alternatives. That is why it is important to ask about them if a radical dissection of the neck is suggested.

Radiation to the neck—
What if you have had it?

For the past two years there has been a bitter controversy about what, if anything, should be done to people who as children were subjected to radiation of the neck in the treatment of benign conditions such as enlarged thymuses, enlarged tonsils, or acne. For more than twenty years it has been known that such radiation often causes nodules to appear in the thyroid and that some of them are papillary cancers. Fortunately, these are almost always so benign that if properly treated, the patients have a normal life expec-

Controversy in
Other Types of Cancer

tancy. Yet many doctors are making mountains out of these thyroid molehills. They are advising everyone who has had radiation to the thyroid to have periodic scans of the thyroid even if the thyroid feels normal. If a scan done with radioactive iodine to show the activity of the thyroid shows anything abnormal, these doctors are advising total *thyroidectomy,* removal of *all* of the thyroid.

Total thyroidectomy would be a perfectly acceptable treatment if that were all that was removed, but the trouble is that too often, all of the parathyroids also are removed. When this happens there is chronic tetany that often is difficult to control.

The incidence of tetany after total thyroidectomy varies with the skill and experience of the surgeon who is operating. Some surgeons claim to have done a hundred or more total thyroidectomies without causing a single case of tetany, whereas others have reported incidences of from 15 percent to 20 percent. I would estimate that in the hands of the ordinary, competent but not specialized surgeon the incidence of tetany would be about 10 percent. It is, therefore, important, if a surgeon wants to perform a *total* thyroidectomy, to ask him how many he has done and what proportion of them had tetany. If this is significant it would be wise to ask him to do a subtotal operation leaving enough capsule to protect the parathyroid on one side, or to find another surgeon who would either do a less than total thyroidectomy or who specialized in thyroid-parathyroid disease and could do the total without significant risk of tetany.

The strange thing about the controversy is that papillary cancer in its early stages is not dangerous. The Mayo Clinic reports that in its entire history, no patient has died of an occult (hidden) papillary cancer such as it takes a scan to find. The life expectancy of the Cleveland Clinic patients with papillary cancer of the thyroid induced by radiation has been normal. Therefore, the wise thing to do, if you have had a history of radiation, is to forget about scans, which only add more radiation to the area, and to have a doctor examine your thyroid once a year. If he finds a lump it is time enough to have the lump removed by removing all of the thyroid on the affected side and almost all of it on the other side. If cancer is present in the specimen, don't worry. If you take thyroid pills for the rest of your life it usually will suppress the growth of any cells that might remain.

General Considerations

We have been dealing thus far with individual cancers and the various methods of treating them. In most types of cancer, radiation and chemotherapy can be used as adjuncts to the primary, surgical treatment. In medical circles the debates about the value of these adjuncts and of the relative value of each type are endless. Many radiologists, for example, believe that radiation given either before or after operations for cancer of the breast greatly reduce the incidence of local recurrence, whereas a distinguished immunologist, Dr. J. R. Stjernsward of Switzerland, has analyzed all the randomized, scientifically controlled trials that have compared the results of surgery alone with those of surgery and radiation and has concluded that in terms of survival there is a small but definite advantage in *not* adding radiation.[6] Since radiation always increases discomfort and disability, I think in the treatment of most kinds of cancer it is best not to use it routinely, but only when there is a definite reason for it, such

Controversy in
Other Types of Cancer

as a strong probability that some of the cancer was not removed.

The value, if any, of giving chemotherapy routinely after operations for cancer is also in question. The hope is that the chemicals will destroy small deposits of cancer cells that have spread throughout the system, whereas they would be ineffective against the metastases if treatment were delayed until metastasis could be seen or felt. At present there is strong evidence both for and against the use of chemotherapy. Its disadvantages are that when given in adequate doses for a year or more, as is often recommended, more than half of the patients lose their hair and are periodically very sick. Also, no one knows if the chemotherapy may of itself cause leukemia or malignancy of the lymphatic system.

In a few years we may be able to say exactly when chemotherapy should or should not be used. In the meantime, I think that in the treatment of most cancers it should be used routinely only in cases in which the cancer has recurred or occasionally in cases in which the outlook for cure by radiation and/or surgery is poor. In addition it should be considered in premenopausal women who have breast cancer with metastasis to nodes and it should be used routinely as an adjuvant at the time of the primary treatment of children with leukemia, lymphomas, malignant tumors of bone, and several other rare, solid tumors in which the value of chemotherapy has been clearly established.

IV

Choices in Nonmalignant Disease

Appendicitis

I am not going to discuss surgical emergencies like *acute appendicitis,* because when you get sick you have no time to shop around. Your decision is whether or not to go ahead with the advice of whoever is there and able to treat you. One point, however, should be made. Do not submit to appendectomy in a substandard hospital or by a substandard surgeon. The peritonitis that appendicitis sometimes causes usually can be prevented or controlled and cured by antibiotics. The risk of a poorly performed appendectomy is greater than that of medical treatment used instead.[1]

As for *chronic appendicitis,* volumes have been written on

Choices in Nonmalignant Disease

this. There was a time when almost every abdominal pain was blamed on this. Then came a time when the existence of chronic appendicitis as a cause of abdominal pain was questioned. I believe the latter position is more nearly correct. Certainly, if the appendix is to be removed in order to relieve chronic pain, the abdomen should be thoroughly explored and certainly, before an operation is done, all other physical and psychological causes should be eliminated, including *fibrositis* of the abdominal wall. The sore, tender area of the abdomen caused by fibrositis is like bursitis and, like bursitis, it is relieved and often cured by injection of hydrocortisone. If you have a tender, painful spot in the abdomen, ask your doctor if it could be a fibrositis and whether injection might bring relief.

Arthritis

The hip is a favorite joint for *arthritis* to attack. This and the constant weight bearing on the joint often cause degeneration of the cartilage that lines the joint. Until recent years such a course of events was a common cause of invalidism, but now the joint can be replaced and the person rehabilitated.

Replacement of the hip is a big operation, and not without danger of complications. In the hands of experts it is highly successful, but it is not an operation that a generalist should do. Be sure to inquire whether your surgeon has made something of a specialty of the operation and is well regarded for his ability in this field. It is not an operation that you would want done by any but the best. The same is true in the

CHOICES IN SURGICAL CARE

replacement of other joints, such as those of the knee, elbow, shoulder, ankle, wrist, or fingers.

Back Pain

I am no authority on back pain. I haven't ever even had one. But one thing I am sure of is that if you have a pain in your back, you should defer surgery and try every other sort of treatment first.

There are exceptions to this rule. If there is evidence that, in spite of conservative treatment, pressure on nerve roots is causing progressive weakness or paralysis of nerves in the legs, it may be well to go straight to surgery before permanent damage is done. But for just a pain in the back, regardless of how severe, try the various conservative treatments first—including rest, traction, injection of steroids, physical therapy, and exercises. Many patients have been helped considerably by one or more of these simple measures or simply by the passage of time.

Most back pain is blamed on "ruptured discs." Discs are the cartilagenous pads between the vertebrae that can rupture and press on nerves. Arthritis, too, can be a cause of pain, with spurs of bone pressing on the nerves. If this is bad enough and the pain can't be controlled, it is possible to fuse the vertebrae together so that the spine can't bend and the nerves aren't compressed. But this is a big, uncomfortable operation that should not be undertaken lightly.

No one knows what causes most pains in the back; hence, there is no universally effective treatment. If x-rays clearly show that there is a ruptured disc, if the pain radiates down

Choices in Nonmalignant Disease

the leg, and if a fair trial of the conservative treatments mentioned above fails, then it is time to try surgery. Even this is not always successful. Time is the greatest healer. Sooner or later most pains in the back subside.

Duodenal Ulcer

Duodenal ulcer is the commonest type of ulcer. It is benign, in that it never turns to cancer, as ulcers in the stomach sometimes do. However, it is common, annoying, and its complications—hemorrhage, obstruction of the outlet of the stomach, or perforation of the bowel causing peritonitis—can be serious or fatal. Fortunately, these complications are rare and can usually be dealt with by operations which entail little greater risk than some of the elective operations that are used in the treatment of uncomplicated ulcer.

Most surgeons agree that the symptoms of duodenal ulcer can, in most cases, be controlled by diet and medicine. The medicine acts to reduce or neutralize the secretion of the stomach's hydrochloric acid. An excess of acid so increases the digestive powers of the gastric juice that it digests the wall of the duodenum (the first part of the small bowel into which the stomach empties its contents). All treatment, medical or surgical, is directed toward reducing or neutralizing the acid. When it is effective, the ulcer heals. When it is not, the ulcer gives pain, especially between meals or at night when there is no food in the stomach to neutralize the acid. ("Drink goat's milk," suggests my wife, Helga Sandburg, life-member of the American Dairy Goat Breeders Association.)

Within the past year there has become available (but still

CHOICES IN SURGICAL CARE

only for limited or experimental use) a powerful drug, Cimetidine, that causes almost complete suppression of the stomach's output of hydrochloric acid. Prompt and complete healing of duodenal ulcers occurs regularly when this drug is given. To date, no serious side effects have been observed, but it is too early to judge its ultimate safety and long-term effectiveness. All that can be said is that it promises to supplant the surgical treatment of duodenal ulcer. For this reason it is important for patients with ulcer to know of this drug so that, if they are not threatened by the complications of hemorrhage, perforation, or obstruction, they can remain on medical treatment and put up with some pain and discomfort until the new treatment becomes generally available.

If a patient with intractable but uncomplicated duodenal ulcer is having so much discomfort that he does not want to wait for the new medical treatment to become available, he has his choice of a variety of operations, each of which is favored by a group of well-qualified surgeons. Each has its advantages and its disadvantages, and each has its risk (mortality rate). In the order of their historic development and rise to popularity they are as follows:

1. Gastroenterostomy alone —obsolete.

Gastric acid is neutralized and short-circuited away from ulcer by joining stomach to a loop of small intestine below the ulcer. Low risk. Few side effects. High rate of recurrence of ulcer.

2. Pyloroplasty alone —obsolete.

Gastric acid is neutralized by widening the pylorus (the outlet of the stomach) so that the alkali from the small intestine can flow back into stomach. Low risk. Few side effects. High rate of recurrence of ulcer.

Choices in Nonmalignant Disease

3. Subtotal gastrectomy alone —still used by some, but nearly obsolete.

Two-thirds or more of the stomach is removed, and the stump is joined to the intestine. High risk (2 percent to 8 percent immediate mortality). Many side effects (loss of weight, vomiting, diarrhea, weakness). Good control of ulcer. Note: *gastric resection* is a general term for removal of part of the stomach, including this operation and antrectomy mentioned below.

4. Vagotomy alone —obsolete.

Cutting of main trunk of the vagus nerve that stimulates the stomach to secrete acid. Low risk. Many side effects, because cutting the vagus nerve paralyzes the stomach and often causes retention of food in stomach, vomiting, and diarrhea. Fair control of duodenal ulcer, but ulcer of stomach sometimes caused by retention of gastric juice in the stomach.

5. Vagotomy and gastroenterostomy —still popular and widely used when the ulcer is causing any obstruction.

The vagus nerve is cut to reduce secretion of acid, and stomach is joined to intestine to enable it to empty. Low risk. Few side effects. About 10 percent chance of new ulcer forming where the stomach is joined to the small intestine.

6. Vagotomy and pyloroplasty —perhaps the most widely done operation today.

The vagus nerve is cut, and outlet of the stomach is widened to allow it to empty. Low risk. Few side effects. About 10 percent chance of recurrence of ulcer.

CHOICES IN SURGICAL CARE

7. Vagotomy and antrectomy —widely used—about as often as vagotomy and pyloroplasty.

The vagus nerve is cut, and the antrum (lower third of the stomach) is removed. Risk about five times as high as that of vagotomy with either pyloroplasty or gastroenterostomy. Fewer side effects than sub-total gastrectomy, but many more than vagotomy with gastroenterostomy or pyloroplasty. Ninety-nine percent complete and permanent control of the ulcer.

8. Selective vagotomy —new operation; rapidly gaining in popularity, but not yet widely used.

Vagus nerve removed from upper part of the stomach where acid is made, and nerve to the lower part of the stomach and intestine left intact so that there is no tendency to diarrhea. Least risk and fewest side effects. Long-term control of ulcer not yet evaluated.

From the above outline of the treatments currently used for controlling duodenal ulcer, it is clear that there is a great deal of difference in the risk (0.2 percent or less for selective vagotomy to 2 percent or more for gastric resection). There are similar differences in the chances of controlling the ulcer (99 percent for vagotomy and antrectomy to 90 percent for vagotomy and pyloroplasty). And there are also differences in the incidence of side effects (20 percent or more for gastric resection to one percent or less for selective vagotomy). In view of this and of the likelihood that there may soon be a medical treatment that will control hitherto intractable ulcers, it would be wise for the patient who has been advised to have an operation for duodenal ulcer to ask his surgeon not only about the various kinds of surgery but also whether it might be safer to wait for the advent of an effective medical treatment than to undergo operation now. If the surgeon

Choices in
Nonmalignant Disease

said the operation was necessary, I would not advise the operation that would be the most likely to cure the ulcer (vagotomy and antrectomy), but the one that had the lowest mortality rate and the lowest incidence of side effects (selective vagotomy or vagotomy and pyloroplasty). If a few years from now the ulcer recurred, in all likelihood it could be treated with the new medicine. This would not be possible if the patient were either dead or disabled from the side effects of a gastric resection.

Gallstones

Until two years ago there was no controversy about the treatment of patients with gallstones that were causing pain, discomfort, or jaundice. Removal of the gallbladder *(cholecystectomy)* was the treatment.

Cholecystectomy is still the treatment for gallstones that are causing severe symptoms, but an experimental treatment involving ingestion of a chemical (chenodyoxycholic acid) promises to dissolve the most common type of gallstones, those composed of cholesterol. It is not yet approved for general use, and shows signs of possibly being toxic in the liver. This treatment is still so new that no one can yet be sure that there are not serious long-range side effects that have not yet come to light. Therefore, if gallstones are causing severe pain, or even more important, if they are causing jaundice, and if the patient is not too old or too fat or too sick, it is still best to remove the gallbladder. The operation is relatively safe (mortality rate about 0.3 percent) and is highly satisfactory in relieving the symptoms. Nevertheless, there is

Choices in Surgical Care

hope that in the future it may be possible to dissolve most gallstones.

The controversy about surgery arises when a person is having no symptoms, but an x-ray taken for some other reason shows gallstones. Here, and in cases where the symptoms are minimal and really not enough to interfere with normal life, there is no agreement as to whether it is better to do nothing or better to remove the stones. Here are the facts and figures:

1. Autopsies on people in their sixties, seventies, and eighties show that about 10 percent of all of them have gallstones. Most of these never caused any symptoms or did any harm. They were not the cause of death nor were they in any way related to it.

2. If the gallstones in 10 percent of the older people in the population had been discovered and removed, even if only 0.3 percent of them died as a result of the operations, that would mean that three in each thousand of the older people of the country would have died of operations designed to protect people from a disease that kills far fewer than that. Thus, if there were ten million people over sixty in the United States, and if all of the ones who had gallstones were operated on, 30,000 would die—not as the result of the gallstones, but as a result of the operations.

Proponents of routinely removing the gallbladder argue that gallstones may be present for years without causing symptoms, but then, when the patient is old and in poor condition, the stones could cause trouble that would necessitate an emergency operation at a time when the patient is so old and sick that the risk of the operation is greatly in-

Choices in Nonmalignant Disease

creased. For this reason, they argue, it is "better to get it over with" while the patient is better able to survive the operation. I am sure that physicians are sincere in this belief, because I know one who had his own symptom-free gallstones removed and know of another surgeon who had the same thing done for his wife.

	Cost	Dis-com-fort	Risk	Side Effects	Possible Complications	Cure
Remove gallbladder	+++	++	+	++	++	++++
No operation	0	0	0*	0*	0*	No symptoms & no cure

*Although there is in the long run a small but definite risk from complications of the stones, the risk from operation is right now whereas the risk from complications is deferred indefinitely. There is thus little question that in terms of life expectancy it is safer not to operate.

There are three fallacies in the kind of reasoning that says, "Let's get it over with now." The first of these is that life is not eternal. For this reason most people with symptom-free gallstones die of other causes before symptoms appear. The second is that if a life is lost from an emergency operation for gallbladder disease done at an advanced age or in the presence of so many other diseases that the patient could not survive the operation, there was not very much pleasant or valuable life sacrificed. The third fallacy, and the important point to remember, is that a gallbladder operation at any age entails a definite risk. For this reason it would be tragic to lose a thirty-five-year-old woman, with the best years of her life ahead of her, as a result of an operation done for a disease that was giving her no trouble and might never trouble her.

CHOICES IN
SURGICAL CARE

Finally, as we said before, there is promise that medical treatments will become available so that all gallstones can be dissolved. This is a case of don't-cross-your-bridge-until-you-come-to-it. By simply waiting you may be able to accomplish the end of removing the stones without an operation.

In balancing the small, future risk of complications from the stones against the small, immediate risk of an operation, one must conclude that when the stones are giving no symptoms it is safer not to operate.

Goiter
(See also Cancer of the Thyroid in Chapter III.)

A goiter is an enlarged thyroid gland. There are several causes. The commonest cause of goiter in some parts of the world, and until 1920 in the Great Lakes and mountainous regions of the United States, was a deficiency of iodine in water and soil. In this country the deficiency has been corrected by adding iodine to table salt.

Now the commonest type of goiter in the United States is a nodule or a number of nodules in the thyroid, often occurring in people who have strong family histories of goiter. This is probably because these families—and the people, mainly women, who get nodules in the thyroid—have some deficiency in the way their thyroid glands make the thyroid hormone. This deficiency stimulates the pituitary gland to secrete a thyroid-stimulating hormone. The hormone not only increases the output of thyroid hormone but also stimu-

Choices in
Nonmalignant Disease

lates the thyroid gland to grow. In the course of this growth lumps of thyroid tissue called *nodules* or *adenomas* appear. These are the common nodular goiters. They can be prevented by giving the patient thyroid hormone, an inexpensive pill made from the thyroid glands of cattle or chemically synthesized, costing only about $10 a year. It causes no side effects. Most thyroid nodules are found by the patient who notices, when he or she looks in the mirror, a little lump in the neck that moves up and down upon swallowing. Sometimes, on a physical examination, the lump is found by the doctor. Then the trouble starts, because the medical profession has something of an obsession about the potential dangers of a nodule in the thyroid.

In Chapter III, we saw that there are several types of cancers of the thyroid, some of which are almost always curable. Others are almost always incurable no matter how early or radically they are treated. The relatively harmless cancers of the thyroid are the common ones; fatal cancers of the thyroid are rare. Cancer of the thyroid is such a rare cause of death, in fact, that in most statistics on death rates from cancer it is not even listed. Cancer of the breast, for example, each year kills more than 40 of each 100,000 people, whereas cancer of the thyroid kills fewer than one. I have often demonstrated this to audiences by asking those who had had a friend or member of the family die of cancer of the thyroid to raise a hand. Usually, in an audience of 200, there will not be a single hand raised. When the same question is asked about cancer of the breast, everyone's hand is up.

Because of the possibility that a nodule in the thyroid is malignant, most physicians do not like to accept the responsibility of treating the small, almost invisible nodule by giving thyroid hormone to suppress its growth. They therefore send the patient to a surgeon. The surgeon has been taught that a thyroid nodule is a potential cancer. Out it comes.

Choices in Surgical Care

The situation with these benign-appearing thyroid nodules is much like the one with symptom-free gallstones: The surgeon is operating to prevent something that might happen. In so doing he subjects the patient to a risk greater than the risk of dying of the thyroid nodule. Since a thyroid nodule is either benign or malignant and rarely, if ever, turns from one to the other, it is clear that the treatment of the nodules has nothing to do with the death rate from the bad kinds of cancers. The dangerous, rapidly growing cancers of the thyroid that cause most of the deaths from thyroid cancer are easily recognized and, even when recognized early, are impossible to cure.

About 5 percent of women over the age of fifty have nodules in their thyroids big enough to be felt. Many more have smaller nodules that can be recognized on scans of the thyroid done with radioactive substances. Almost all people of this age have microscopic nodules in their thyroids. If the pathologist looks hard enough and cuts many sections, he can find microscopic cancer in anywhere from 5 percent to 20 percent of the supposedly normal thyroids. But this is the kind of microscopic in-situ cancer or "pathologist's cancer" that is not recognized clinically, causes no symptoms, and rarely turns into true cancer. It is like the "cancer" of the prostate that occurs in 35 percent of all men over age fifty, as discussed in Chapter III.

Although these microscopic cancers of the thyroid cannot be recognized clinically, most of the true cancers can be— not only the "bad" ones that were mentioned before, constituting about 15 percent of all thyroid cancers, but also the "good" ones—the papillary cancers that constitute 70 percent of all cancers of the thyroid. About half of these papillary cancers spread to the lymph nodes of the neck so that they can be felt there and malignancy can be suspected. About half of the rest of the papillary cancers infiltrate the gland

Choices in
Nonmalignant Disease

and are so hard that an experienced examiner can make the diagnosis by touch. These and the ones with involved nodes should be removed.

But what about the vast majority of thyroid nodules that are small, give no symptoms, are of no cosmetic importance, and are discovered only by accident? These are the ones over which there is controversy. The following are the diverse points of view.

Many surgeons of the old school believe that all thyroid nodules should be removed. Let us assume that there are 100,000,000 adults in this country and that 5 percent of them have detectable nodules in their thyroids. Let us further suppose that all of this 5 percent (5,000,000 people) have their thyroids removed. The operation is relatively safe, but fatal accidents during anesthesia or postoperatively, by choking from sudden hemorrhage, can and do occur in perhaps one operation in 1,000. That would mean that 5,000 lives would be lost in operations designed to cure a disease that in all of its forms would cause only 1,000 deaths in the original 100,000,000 adults. Moreover, most of the deaths from thyroid cancer occur in the small group of patients who have rapidly growing cancers, and whom the operation would not cure in any case. Finally, the deaths that occur from operations occur right now, whereas deaths that occur as a result of the kind of slowly growing thyroid cancer that could not be recognized clinically would not be apt to take place for ten to twenty years.

The majority of surgeons now believe that the only nodules that should be operated on are those that raise the possibility of cancer because of the age (youth) of the patient, a history of having been exposed as a child to radiation of the neck, the sex (male) of the patient, or the consistency (hardness) of the nodule. The rest can be treated by suppressive doses of thy-

Choices in Surgical Care

roid hormone which prevents them from enlarging and sometimes causes them to shrink.

Some surgeons, in recent years, have taken up what has been standard practice in European clinics for two decades: only those nodules in which a clinical diagnosis of cancer is suspected are removed. The rest have a *needle biopsy* made in the office. The neck is anesthetized with a drop of novocaine and an empty, ordinary hypodermic needle is inserted into the nodule. Pulling up the plunger as the needle point is moved back and forth sucks cellular material into the syringe. The sucked-up material is then put in a fixative solution. The pathologist takes the cellular sediment from the bottom of the jar, makes a cell block of it, and studies it with a microscope. In more than 80 percent of the cases, he can predict accurately that no cancer is present. These patients do not require operation and can be treated by feeding thyroid hormone. The rest require operations, and only about a third of them are found to have cancer. More than 80 percent of the patients are thus spared operation. A special dividend is that in 30 percent of the cases, the nodules are cysts filled with fluid, many of which disappear and never come back.

Surgeons in this country have been slow to take up needle biopsy of the thyroid. There is nothing new about it. It has been practiced widely in Scandinavia, Switzerland, and France for more than twenty years, and has been used and described in professional journals by surgeons and pathologists at the Massachusetts General Hospital, Memorial Hospital in New York, and the Cleveland Clinic. In many parts of the country, however, pathologists have been slow to use the technique of making diagnoses from small clusters of cells obtained by needle biopsy, and this, in turn, has prevented surgeons from adopting this approach. In the meantime,

Choices in Nonmalignant Disease

thousands of harmless nodules of the thyroid are removed each year.

	Cost	Dis-com-fort	Risk	Side Effects	Possible Complications	Survival
Routine removal of nodules	+++++	++	++	++	++	Same*
Selective removal of nodules	++	+	+	+	+	Same
Needle biopsy of all benign-appearing nodules	+	0+	0+	0+	0+	Same

*Not as high if mortality rate of the operation itself is considered.

If the surgeon suspects that you have cancer of the thyroid and wishes to operate, be sure to ask him if he is going to remove all of the thyroid or only most of it. This is important because, as discussed under "Cancer of the Thyroid" in Chapter III, total removal is apt to cause tetany, a permanent lowering of blood calcium due to accidental removal of the parathyroids. It might also be well to ask your surgeon how many total thyroidectomies he has done and what proportion of his patients have had permanent tetany. This advice is pertinent only when the surgeon intends to perform a *total* thyroidectomy.

CHOICES IN
SURGICAL CARE

Heart Disease
(Coronary Bypass Surgery)

Coronary bypass operations are still somewhat controversial, some cardiologists believing that they have been accepted with too much enthusiasm and that too many of them are being done. Many of the operations are done because the patients are suffering the pains of *angina pectoris,* a symptom of blockage of the coronary artery that brings blood to the muscle of the heart. Most patients with angina are relieved of their pain by the bypass operation. But what effect does the operation have on their life expectancies? This depends on the mortality rate of the operation in the hospital where it is done. It depends also on the number of arteries that are blocked.

In a series of such operations done at the Cleveland Clinic, when only one vessel was bypassed, the mortality rate of the operation was less than 2 percent. This mortality, however, is enough to neutralize any gain in survival that the bypass might give to a person with a minimally damaged heart. Therefore, if the pain is not severe and only one vessel is affected, there is no use having the operation.

If two or three arteries are blocked, requiring multiple bypasses, the operative mortality is increased to as much as 4 percent—but these patients, if left untreated, die of their disease at such a rate that the operation gives them a striking benefit in survival. However, if the mortality rate at a particular hospital reaches 10 percent, the advantage has vanished. The recently reported mortality rates in various hospitals in one large city varied by a factor of 5 (that is to say, the risk of dying of the operation was five times as high in some hospitals as in others), so it is obvi-

Choices in Nonmalignant Disease

ous that the patients who were subjected to operations in the high-risk hospitals would have been safer without an operation.

The authors of a recent article on coronary bypass operations done at the Veterans Administration Hospitals concluded that the operations did not appear to prolong the lives of the patients.[2] Critics, however, were quick to point out that the reason that lives were not prolonged was that the surgeons performing the operations had high mortality rates that canceled out any increase in life expectancy that the bypass might have given.[3] Again it seems that it is not so much a question whether the operation is good for the disease but rather whether the surgeon can perform the operation safely.

Hemorrhoids

Hemorrhoids are varicose veins in the anal area. Those in the upper part are called *internal*. Those low in the anal canal are called *external*. For more than a century *hemorrhoidectomy*—cutting out the hemorrhoids and an adjacent section of the skin—was the only way to get rid of these troublesome enlargements of the veins. The operation was done under anesthesia, and it meant several days of hospitalization, a great deal of discomfort, and pain with bowel movements for two weeks or more, until the area was healed. It was an operation that most people dreaded. An occasional complication is *stricture*, or narrowing of the anus.

Several years ago an enterprising innovator devised the

CHOICES IN SURGICAL CARE

rubber-band technique of hemorrhoidectomy. It is done in the office, requires no anesthesia, and rarely causes significant pain. This treatment is suitable for all uncomplicated cases of internal hemorrhoids. External hemorrhoid tabs are not often troublesome, but when they are they can be dealt with by simply excising them.

	Cost	Discomfort	Risk	Side Effects	Possible Complications	Cure
Hemorrhoidectomy	+++	+++	0+	+	Stricture	Same
Rubber Band	+	0+	0	0	0	Same*

*Cure of internal hemorrhoids is excellent but external tabs may require separate attention.

The operation takes advantage of the fact that there is no sensation of pain in the mucous membrane that covers the upper parts of the hemorrhoidal veins. The dilated vein is exposed through a proctoscope, grasped with a special instrument, and pulled up so that a rubber band, provided by the same instrument, can be snapped over the hemorrhoid. This cuts off the circulation to the banded tissue; in a few days it sloughs away, the rubber band falls off, and the wound heals over. The entire procedure is practically painless, takes only a few minutes, requires no hospitalization, and effectively removes the venous part of the hemorrhoid, which in most cases is the troublesome part. In spite of this some surgeons still routinely employ the standard nineteenth-century hemorrhoidectomy. That is why, if you have hemorrhoids, it is important to find out what alternatives there are to the conventional operation.

Choices in Nonmalignant Disease

Hernia Repair

The repair of an ordinary *inguinal* (groin) *hernia* in a child or in an adult who is in good health is an operation that is simple, effective, and done well by most general surgeons. It is the operation that interns and residents cut their teeth on. If you are not overweight, you don't have to worry too much about who does the operation. What you should look into is whether the operation needs to be done.

Many men have a relaxation of the ring through which the cord to the testicles enters the abdomen and through which the contents of the abdominal cavity tend to bulge. When this is well defined, visible, palpable, and uncomfortable, it is called a *direct inguinal hernia,* and should be repaired. When it is small, invisible, and causes no symptoms it is called a *relaxed inguinal ring.* Since this does not necessarily progress to a true hernia it requires no treatment. If it begins to be uncomfortable, then it is time enough to have it repaired. There is absolutely no danger in having such a weakness and no advantage in having it repaired. Unfortunately, however, some employers demand a pre-employment physical examination, and if such a weakness is found they may deny you employment on the grounds that if a true hernia did develop they would be responsible. This state of affairs results in many unnecessary operations.

The commonest type of hernia, occurring in both men and women, but mostly in men, is the *indirect inguinal hernia.* This type is the result of a birth defect in which the peritoneum that lines the abdominal cavity continues on down into the scrotum and sometimes around the testicle, or, in the case of women, into the labia. This, coupled with a defect in the abdominal wall, makes it possible for abdominal fat or a loop of bowel to descend into the sac. Sometimes it can get stuck there (impacted) so that it cannot return to the abdomen. This calls for an immediate operation before the blood supply of the bowel is affected, which would risk potentially fatal gangrene and intestinal obstruction. Since patients with large indirect inguinal hernias often have such complications, it is wise to have such a hernia repaired before symptoms occur.

If you are much overweight, and especially if the hernia is a large direct one, it might be well to select a surgeon who has made something of a specialty of operating for hernias. The same is true of a hernia that has recurred after an unsuccessful operation. Special help should also be obtained if you are overweight and have a recurrent hernia in the scar of an abdominal operation.

In almost every community there is a surgeon who makes a subspecialty of hernia operations. If your problem is one of the complicated ones listed above, you would do well to ask your family doctor or a surgeon friend whom to go to. There is, in fact, one medical group composed of several surgeons at the Shouldice Clinic in Toronto who do nothing but hernia operations. Most of these are done under local anesthesia, and the patient leaves the hospital in one to three days.

Hyperthyroidism

Overactivity of the thyroid *(hyperthyroidism)* causes nervousness, rapid pulse, tremor, sweating, and loss of weight. It can be caused by overactivity of the nodules in a large *goiter* (see earlier this chapter). In that case almost everyone agrees

Choices in
Nonmalignant Disease

that the best treatment is to remove most of the thyroid. The other and by far the most common type of hyperthyroidism is called *Graves' disease*— a condition in which there are no nodules, all of the gland is overactive, and sometimes there is no enlargement of the thyroid, so that it is referred to as an "inward goiter." There is controversy about whether to treat this type of goiter by removing it or by giving radioactive iodine. Naturally enough, most surgeons say operate, and radiologists (who administer the radioactive iodine) say it is best to treat with radioactive iodine. Here are the pros and cons.

Those who favor radioactive iodine point out that it entails no risk of death and has no side effects except *hypothyroidism*, the easily corrected deficiency of thyroid. Treatment of Graves' disease with radioactive iodine involves no hospitalization, no discomfort, and no scar or risk of permanent injury to the function of the vocal cords or the parathyroid glands. It permanently controls the hyperthyroidism in more than 99 percent of the cases, and if there is recurrence it can be retreated. It has been in use for more than thirty years. Hundreds of thousands of patients have been treated, and extensive studies have shown no increase in cancer of the thyroid, of cancer elsewhere in the body, of leukemia, or of hereditary defects in the children of treated people. In short, it seems to be as close to the ideal treatment as can be found. The one defect, the production of hypothyroidism, is corrected at the cost of $10 a year for thyroid tablets taken from the time that the hyperthyroidism is controlled. No medical checkups are needed so long as the patient takes the prescribed replacement dose of thyroid once a day.

Some physicians still hesitate to treat children with radioactive iodine, but in the more than thirty years' experience there have been no side effects other than the easily corrected hypothyroidism.

Choices in
Surgical Care

The thyroid cells are radiated so intensively by treatment with radioactive iodine that they not only cannot function, they also cannot divide. The situation is totally different from the cases in which the thyroid is given a small dose of radiation and the cells can still reproduce. After the large dose the cells are sterilized. A cell that cannot divide cannot give rise to a cancer. Radioactive iodine, therefore, does not increase the possibility of getting cancer of the thyroid; it actually protects against it.

In spite of this widespread knowledge, as recently as May 1977, a friend of mine, a woman attorney who held a responsible public position, was advised by an endocrinologist to have a thyroidectomy for Graves' disease. There were no nodules and no specific indications for surgery. During the operation, the recurrent laryngeal nerve, which controls the function of the vocal cords, was damaged. She woke up hoarse, and has been so since, with no ability to project her voice. This, occurring in a lawyer in mid-career, has been a severe blow. "The doctor told me that the radioactive iodine might cause cancer," she explained to me. "I simply didn't double-check it."

Opposition to the use of radioactive iodine is rapidly fading, not so much because the surgeons have changed their minds and prefer not to operate, but rather because most of the diagnosing physicians no longer send their patients to the surgeons, but have them treated with radioactive iodine instead. Then, too, this is what the patients prefer, with the result that many of them simply refuse surgery and seek out the other treatment. That is why, if thyroidectomy is suggested as the treatment of an overactive thyroid, you should ask about alternatives or get a second opinion. This applies to children as well as older people because experience has shown that there are no disadvantages to treating children with radioactive iodine. It applies to the most common type

Choices in Nonmalignant Disease

of hyperthyroidism associated with Graves' disease, but not to all patients with nodular goiter and hyperthyroidism. The following chart compares the results of the two treatments of hyperthyroidism associated with Graves' disease.

	Cost	Dis-com-fort	Risk	Side Effects	Possible Complications	Cure
Removal of the thyroid	+ ++	+ ++	++	Scar	Tetany, vocal cord paralysis, hypothyroidism	90% (Depends on how much removed)
Radioactive iodine	++	0	0	0	Hypothyroidism (more than with Thyroidectomy but easily controlled)	99+%

Ingrown Toenails

Standard advice to patients with painful *ingrown toenails* is to cut them square in the hopes that this will prevent the ingrowth of the edges of the nail. This is fine if the nail is not causing much discomfort, but in my experience it never helps the bad cases. Although for these, many surgeons advise removing the nails, I have found that this is not often necessary. Instead, the patient should buy a pair of strong nail clippers and he himself, in spite of some discomfort, should cut out the corners of the ingrown nails right down to the quick. This should be repeated periodically. It gets easier with experience, and after each treatment the toes are perfectly comfortable until the nails grow back.

Lipomas

A *lipoma* is a benign tumor of fat. It grows slowly, does not tend to become malignant, and does not need to be removed unless it gets big enough to be conspicuous or uncomfortable. Some people have many of them under the skin, all over the body, arms, and legs. They can be diagnosed accurately by their softness.

Most lipomas can be removed easily under local anesthesia in the office or in out-patient surgery. If the tumor is in a place where a long scar would be conspicuous, a very small incision can be made into the tumor and its soft contents squeezed until they plop out, capsule and all. The same small-incision technique can be used to remove *sebaceous cysts* (wens) of the scalp or elsewhere on the body.

Pilonidal Cyst or Sinus

The acute abscesses that occur over the tailbone are called *pilonidal cysts*. The open, draining sinuses that occur in the same area are called *pilonidal sinuses*. *Pilo* means "hair" and *nid* means "nest"; these are "hair nest" diseases. They are of

Choices in
Nonmalignant Disease

special interest because, of all of the absurd overtreatments that through the centuries surgeons have devised, the prime example is the operation for pilonidal disease.

Pilonidal disease is the result of ingrown hairs. In hairy persons the cleft between the buttocks directs the hairs downward toward the little depression that many people have just at the tip of the tailbone where, in the development of the embryo, the nervous system turned in from the skin. The hairs penetrate the skin of this tender area and embed themselves in the tissues, where they fester, causing abscesses or draining sinuses. Sometimes there are only a few hairs and sometimes there is a large collection, forming a sort of hair ball. All that needs to be done is to have the hair removed. Often it can be done in the office, under local anesthesia, by opening the abscess and inserting a little rubber tube which is anchored in place for two or three weeks until the hairs have been extruded and the cavity has filled in. The tube is then withdrawn, the buttocks are shaved or treated with a depilatory to remove all hair, and the area is soon healed. In the case of a draining sinus, the hairs that cause the trouble often can be removed by scraping out the tract with a little crochet hook. Again the buttocks are shaved and usually the sinus heals up. When it doesn't it can be opened by a minor operation and scraped clean of all hair.

But what is the standard operation done in hospitals throughout the country? The standard operation for pilonidal cyst or sinus is to *cut the whole thing out* just as if it were a cancer. Since the area is infected, healing is slow. Often the surgeon doesn't shave the buttocks, with the result that the irritation from the hair as the patient walks keeps scraping the wound open so that it never heals. Then the surgeon admits the patient for a skin graft. Often a week or more of hospitalization is involved, as

Choices in
Surgical Care

well as the discomfort of a large operation in a sore place.

Why do surgeons do all this when the disease is so easily cured by a simple office treatment? The question is impossible to answer, except in terms of economics and habit.

A century ago when pilonidal disease was first described by an English surgeon, he noted that by looking closely the hair could be seen growing *into* it from without. Then someone else described a congenital misplacement of tissue in the pelvis that causes what is known as a *presacral dermoid* (skinlike) *cyst* that contains skin, hair, and teeth. Very, very rarely, one of these drains externally from the same area as a pilonidal sinus. The dermoid cyst, of course, has to be removed, because hair follicles are growing within it, whereas pilonidal disease can be treated by simply removing the hair that grows into it from without. Somehow the two conditions got confused in the minds of surgeons and of teachers in medical schools, so that removal of the whole cyst or sinus became standard practice for the treatment of ingrown hairs.

In the 1940s, studies were made by surgeons and pathologists that showed beyond doubt that there were no hair roots or follicles in pilonidal abscesses or sinuses. Undeterred, surgeons kept on cutting them out to get rid of the last nonexistent root.

Pilonidal cysts or sinuses affect young men. The condition is aggravated by bumpy riding—it was called "jeep disease" in World War II. Radical operations done for this disease caused more prolonged disability than any other surgical condition at the San Diego Naval Hospital. When I worked there, there was always a ward full of pilonidal convalescents. Some of them took a year to heal.

You can't blame fee-for-service surgery for the radical pilonidal operations that were done on military personnel during the war. It is the teaching that must get the blame. This in

Choices in Nonmalignant Disease

turn may have been influenced by the fee-for-service system, because it is surgeons who teach surgery, and most of them get their income from fee-for-service surgery. (See discussion of this problem in Part Two.) There would be little incentive for them to switch from an operation for which they get paid hundreds of dollars to a simple office treatment for which they get paid very little. It would also be impossible for a teacher of surgery to teach a treatment he was not practicing. Hence, even though the true nature and proper treatment of pilonidal disease has been known for more than thirty years, radical surgery still is the most commonly recommended treatment. Please, if anyone wants to hospitalize you for an operation for previously untreated pilonidal disease, refuse the operation and go looking for another surgeon!

Polyps

Polyps are small, benign growths that grow, many of them like cherries on stalks, from the lining of the colon and rectum. The ones in the lower part of the colon or in the rectum can be seen and removed through a sigmoidoscope or proctoscope. Now the colonoscope makes it possible to remove them throughout the entire colon. (These instruments are lighted, flexible tubes inserted into the rectum, through which the lining of the colon and rectum can be viewed.)

A polyp may bleed, but aside from that it gives no symptoms. Most of them are discovered either on proctoscopic examination or on an x-ray of the colon. Concern about them is based upon the fact that some of them show early malig-

CHOICES IN
SURGICAL CARE

nant change—in-situ, noninvasive cancer, like that discussed under "Cancer of the Cervix" in Chapter III—and others, the kind without stalks, may have true cancers that invade. The cancer is harmless so long as it does not invade the stalk of the polyp or its base. All that need be done is to have the polyp removed and the base cauterized through the proctoscope or colonoscope. Yet, until recently, and still in some parts of the country, there are surgeons so radical that when there is a malignant polyp they advise removal of the affected segment of the colon or rectum, an operation that carries with it a 2 percent to 5 percent mortality rate. This makes the danger of operation much greater than the danger of the cancer. When an abdominal operation for a polyp is suggested, therefore, it is wise to ask about alternatives. Remember, it is now possible in most cases to remove polyps *anywhere* in the colon by colonoscopy. If cancer can be shown to be invading the polyp's base, the affected part of the colon can then be removed.

	Cost	Discomfort	Risk	Side Effects	Possible Complications	Survival
Removing part of colon	+ ++	+ ++	+ ++	+ ++	+ ++	Same
Removing polyp	+	0+	0+	0	0	Same

[94]

Choices in
Nonmalignant Disease

Prostate Gland—Benign Enlargement
(See also Cancer of the Prostate Gland
in Chapter III.)

In order to equalize the burdens of the sexes, women were born with uteri and men with prostate glands. If a man lives a long time he is as apt to have something go wrong with his prostate as a woman is with her uterus.

The commonest disorder of the prostate is *benign hypertrophy*—a lumpy type of growth that is not malignant but which presses on the outlet of the urinary bladder and interferes with urination. Most men beyond the age of sixty-five have some degree of urinary obstruction. Some have complete retention, in which they can't urinate at all, and have to have a rubber catheter inserted through the penis to empty the bladder. Often an emergency operation is necessary. For most men, however, the condition goes on for years with little progress. There is the embarrassment of taking a long time to urinate and that of dribbling or of occasional incontinence of urine. The majority, however, learn to live with their problem and die of other causes before an operation on the prostate is necessary.

The treatment for obstruction by a benign enlargement of the prostate depends on the severity of the symptoms, on their response to medical treatment, on the size of the gland, on the age and well-being of the patient, and on the special skills of the surgeon. If the symptoms are mild and consist only of having to get up a couple of times a night or of a little dribbling after urination, all that usually is necessary is to have a urologist examine the prostate (a rectal examination) to see if there is any evidence of malignancy. If not, and if there is no sign of retention of urine, no treatment is necessary. On the other hand, if a large amount of urine is retained

Choices in Surgical Care

in the bladder after urination, or if the bladder and the ureters, which carry the urine from kidneys to bladder, are dilated from back pressure, it is best to have an operation.

Sometimes enlargement of the prostate results in irritability of the bladder and in spasm, causing frequency and urgency of urination and occasionally even involuntary urination. Appropriate medicines can do much to control these symptoms and sometimes enable the patient to avoid operation.

When the gland is very large the surgeon may feel that it is better to remove it by an abdominal operation called *suprapubic prostatectomy*. This is somewhat more uncomfortable and entails a higher risk of complications, including fatality, than does the operation done from below through an instrument inserted into the urethra. The latter is called *transurethral resection*, and involves cutting out the part of the gland that blocks the urethra. Since this requires special training and skill, it would be wise to investigate the surgeon's training qualifications and experience before accepting a transurethral resection. If the gland is very large and the patient relatively young, the larger suprapubic prostatectomy may give a better and more lasting result.

The following table evaluates both types of treatment available for enlargement of the prostate.

	Cost	Discomfort	Risk	Side Effects	Possible Complications	Cure
Transurethral resection	+++	++	+	+	+	Same*
Suprapubic prostatectomy	+++	+++	++	++	++	Same

*In some, operations may have to be repeated.

Choices in Nonmalignant Disease

Occasionally, when an enlarged prostate is removed or resected, a microscopic area of cancer is found in the specimen. As mentioned in the section on Cancer of the Prostate Gland, such microscopic cancers are present in the prostate glands of nearly half of all older men. In spite of this they do not often grow into true, trouble-making cancers. For this reason, it is not always necessary to have radical treatment by surgery, radiation, or endocrine therapy. The side effects are too great. It is often wiser to do nothing and to wait and see if trouble comes. If it does, there is still plenty of time to treat it.

Tonsillectomy and Adenoidectomy

Tonsillectomy has come in for much criticism as an unnecessary operation, yet many unnecessary tonsillectomies are still being done. Most of these, however, are not done by qualified *otolaryngologists* (ear, nose, and throat experts) but by general practitioners or general surgeons. Most tonsillectomies are not only unnecessary but also undesirable. All operations carry a risk, and tonsillectomy is no exception. A number of children still die each year as a result of this operation.

Tonsillectomies are justified under certain limited circumstances. When a child, or a person of any age, gets a series of abscesses in the tissues behind the tonsil, proved by repeated cultures, tonsillectomy may be the best way to stop them. If the tonsils are so large that they block the airway, it is possible that the lungs and ultimately the heart will be damaged. This situation is exceedingly rare but is corrected at once by tonsillectomy.

Adenoids are apt to give more trouble than tonsils because they may block the air tube in the ear and impair hearing. When they do they should be removed. Since the operations of tonsillectomy and *adenoidectomy* still are being done much more often than necessary, it is best, when there is the least doubt, to ask for a second opinion. If a pediatrician has suggested the operation, ask another pediatrician. If a general practitioner or general surgeon has suggested it, ask both a pediatrician and an ear, nose, and throat specialist.

Vaginal Repair Operations

Gynecologists are experienced in repairing the relaxations of the front or back vaginal wall that can follow childbirth and result in the bladder or rectum pushing the vaginal walls downward and finally out of the vagina. In addition the uterus may *prolapse*—that is to say, slide down through the vagina and protrude from it. These conditions are like hernias in that they are induced by gravity pushing the abdominal contents down through a weak spot in the pelvic muscles. Gynecologists usually are far better trained in repairing these defects than general surgeons, and usually do it with excellent results and few complications. Operations, however, can result in scarring or vaginal shortening since new tissue is not grafted in to replace the old. Remember, these operations are completely optional; you, not the surgeon, should decide to have the operation done. You do not

Choices in Nonmalignant Disease

need to have it unless you are uncomfortable. Nothing is gained by having the operation done at once instead of later and no complications are avoided by an early operation.

There is one exception to the above statments. If the weakness is in the front wall, resulting in inability to control the flow of urine, it would be wise to consult a urologist as well as a gynecologist. This condition may or may not require surgical treatment. Incontinence is a great nuisance, and for best results the operation should be done by a surgeon who has made it something of a subspecialty.

Varicose Veins

Varicose veins are extremely common and usually are of little consequence. They tend to run in families, and to be made worse by standing still. Exercise, on the other hand, is good for them. That is because the cause of the varicosities is defective valves in the veins of the legs. These fail to check the column of blood that flows into the legs' veins all the way to the heart, so that when the patient stands, the pressure of the column distends the veins. The motion of walking, on the other hand, tends to pump the blood out of the veins and back up to the heart.

When varicose veins are large they can damage the circulation, leading to painful ulcers at the ankle. They can also be the site of clots—*thromboses* that get sore and occasionally can be swept by the bloodstream to the lungs, causing an embolism. This complication, however, is rare. The main reason for treating varicose veins is to improve the appearance of the legs and to make them more comfortable.

CHOICES IN SURGICAL CARE

There are two methods of treating varicose veins. One is by *ligation* (tying off) of the vein and removing it by *stripping* it out with a special instrument. After this the blood returns to the heart satisfactorily through the deep veins. This operation is very safe and effective, but over a period of years varicosities may appear in other veins. The other method of treatment is by *injection* with a fluid that irritates the walls of the vein. A compression bandage is then applied for several weeks until the vein has sealed itself off and blood cannot enter it. This method is effectively used in England and in some centers in the United States. Its disadvantage is that one has to wear a cumbersome pressure bandage for several weeks. If this method is elected, one should seek out a physician who has had special experience or training in using it.

Vascular Surgery

In the last twenty years remarkable strides have been made in *vascular surgery*—operations on the blood vessels. No artery is now out of reach of the surgeon, from the huge *aorta* that carries all the blood from the heart, to the small *coronary arteries* of the heart itself. (See section on Heart Disease.) All of them, including those that nourish the brain as well as those of the legs, can now be cleaned out or replaced by grafts. The risk is high or low depending on the location and severity of the disease and on the skill of the surgeon. Today, patients who years ago invariably would have died of rupture of an *aneurysm* (pulsating swelling) of the aorta, now live comfortably after removal and insertion of a graft. Often,

Choices in
Nonmalignant Disease

strokes can be avoided by paying heed to small symptoms. This leads to tests showing obstruction to vessels of the brain and to removal of the clots that are blocking those vessels. All of this should be done by surgeons who have had special training in vascular surgery or who limit their practice to vascular surgery. The risk of operation will be much higher in the hands of a general surgeon who only occasionally operates on arteries, than in the hands of a specialist. In most communities there are medical specialists who do not operate but treat vascular disease, and it would be to one of these that I would go for advice about which vascular surgeon to see.

V

Annual Checkup and the Diagnosis of Surgical Problems

In diagnosis, as well as in treatment, there are many areas of controversy. One of the most important is whether money spent on periodic medical checkups, such as the "annual physical examination," is a sound investment for a person who feels well. Or is it merely an expensive way of soothing anxiety? "It finds too little and it costs too much," argues Dr. Richard Spark of the Harvard Medical School, and I agree.[1]

Annual Checkup and the Diagnosis of Surgical Problems

The Complete Physical

Consider the physical examination of a person who has no symptoms at all, and let's see what abnormalities might be found and whether finding them could be expected to prolong either life or health.

1. Eyes. One disorder that can be found in the eyes is glaucoma, an increased pressure in the fluid chamber of the eye that can cause damage to the retina and result in a gradual loss of vision. Since any vision that is lost to glaucoma cannot be recovered and since effective medical and surgical remedies for the increased pressure are available, it is worthwhile for persons over the age of forty to have their eyes tested for glaucoma every few years. However, you are not apt to get this test because the examination for glaucoma is not often done by the internists who do annual physical examinations. It is done routinely in eye examinations by ophthalmologists and many opticians also are equipped with the special instruments required to do the test.

Glaucoma is the only disorder of the eye in which there is an advantage in treating the disease before it causes symptoms. Cataracts, detached retinas, and other common diseases of the eye result in loss of vision that the patient recognizes. There is no hurry about the treatment of cataracts, but when loss of vision is due to a detached retina it should be treated promptly before it progresses and more vision is lost.

Any loss of vision is, of course, a sign that you should have an eye examination. A sudden but transitory loss of vision in one eye is a clear indication for an examination by a neurologist or by an internist interested in diseases

Choices in Surgical Care

of the blood vessels. The temporary loss of vision could indicate partial blockage of an artery and could be a forerunner of a stroke. If recognized and treated, the blockage can be removed and the stroke avoided. But here again we are not talking about a patient who has no symptoms. We are talking about one who has had some loss of vision, even if transitory. That is why any new symptom should be reported to your doctor. But if you have no symptom, why go?

Perhaps when you hit middle age and begin to get so farsighted that your arms aren't long enough to hold the telephone book where you can read it, it is a good thing to have an eye examination. But if you never before have had to wear glasses, don't let anyone talk you into prescription lenses. At the dime store for a tenth the price you can fit yourself to standard magnifiers that will help you just as much. They have nice frames and look well, too.

2. Ears. There is no disease of the ear that when treated early gives more satisfactory results than when treated after symptoms are present.

3. Nose and Throat. Most cancers of the nose, mouth, throat, and larynx give symptoms early enough so that if hoarseness or discomfort are reported promptly there will be as good a chance of cure as there would be if an unspecialized physician had looked at these organs once a year.

4. Neck. The neck contains many lymph nodes which may swell up when there are infections of the throat or may be enlarged as a result of cancer. Usually these are noticed by the patient about as early as they can be felt

Annual Checkup and the Diagnosis of Surgical Problems

by the physician. The same is true of nodules in the thyroid. Of course, any persistent nodes or nodules should be examined by your doctor.

5. Lungs. It would be most unusual for a physician to find, on physical examination or by listening with a stethoscope, any disease of the lungs that gave no cough at all and no symptoms of pain, wheezing, or shortness of breath. In a person with no symptoms at all, even x-ray of the chest rarely shows anything in the lung at a stage where treatment would be more successful than if given later. For example, in a ten-year study of more than 6,000 men who smoked cigarettes, x-rays of the chest were taken twice a year. Of the 121 who were found to have cancers of the lung, obviously detected at about as early a stage as possible, only 8 percent lived five years, the same proportion as in patients whose symptoms had led them to examination.[2]

There is a definite advantage to diagnosing tuberculosis early, but usually even early tuberculosis gives symptoms, and fortunately, in recent years, tuberculosis has become so rare that the Tuberculosis Society is no longer recommending routine chest x-rays.

6. Abdomen. If a person were a heavy drinker it might be well to have a physician feel the abdomen once a year to see if the liver were enlarged by fat or hardened by cirrhosis, but the kind of person who drinks that much would not be apt to consult a physician. I can think of no other finding in the abdomen that in the absence of any symptoms would be apt to lead to life-saving treatment.

7. Genitalia. Men usually are conscious of any changes in the genitalia. Women, on the other hand, may have early cancer of the cervix without having any symptoms at all. This can be diagnosed by the Pap test and treated while still curable. Sexually active women beyond the age of twenty should have Pap smears taken every two or three years even if they have no symptoms. The likelihood of cervical cancer is higher in women whose sexual activity started when young. Other cancers of the uterus cause abnormal bleeding, which of course should always be reported.

Ovarian cancer can be detected on pelvic examination, but it is so rare that the chance of having one accidentally detected on a routine pelvic examination is low. Nevertheless, it is worthwhile having the pelvis examined at the time the Pap smear is taken.

8. Breasts. Examination of the breasts is best done by the patient herself, and from the age of thirty on should be done once a month. Mammograms every five years after the age of forty are of value in detecting cancers too small to be felt. After the age of fifty, mammograms can be taken every two or three years without danger of overexposure to radiation.

9. Rectum. In the male a rectal examination may reveal an enlarged prostate, but if this is causing no symptoms there is no use knowing about it. It can be treated satisfactorily after symptoms are present.

It is conceivable that a cancer of the rectum could be found on rectal examination, but almost certainly, if the patient has taken the common-sense precaution of looking at all his stools, he or she would have seen blood or mucus and would have reported it to the doctor.

Annual Checkup and the Diagnosis of Surgical Problems

10. Proctoscopic examination. Most physicians do not have equipment for doing a satisfactory proctoscopic examination but they may refer the patient to a specialist. Here again, if the patient had had no blood in the stool it is rare that anything significant would be found. Benign polyps may be present and these can be burned off, but there is no proof that these would ever have caused trouble if left alone. Nevertheless, a proctoscopic examination done by a competent examiner or specialist once in every four or five years might pick up an occasional polyp with early malignant change. Considering the discomfort and expense of the examination it is doubtful that it should be done as often as once a year. People with a family history of cancer of the bowel should be examined more often.

11. Nervous system. In a person with no symptoms, there is no disease of the nervous system that can be found on physical examination at a time when there is an advantage in treating it right away.

12. Heart and blood pressure. There is a definite advantage in recognizing the presence of high blood pressure and, if it is excessively high, in treating it early. In this way the complications of high blood pressure, stroke, heart disease, and kidney failure can be postponed or avoided. If you want to, you can buy the inexpensive instrument and learn to take your own pressure and those of your family and friends.

There is nothing helpful that can be found by listening to the heart of a person who has no symptoms at all. Of course, if there is pain in the chest, shortness of breath, or swelling of the ankles, these symptoms of heart disease should be reported. The electrocardiogram, unfor-

Choices in Surgical Care

tunately, tells us what has already happened to the heart rather than what is going to happen.

After surveying the benefits of the complete physical examination we have come up with the facts that the eyes of older people should be tested for glaucoma every four or five years, that a Pap smear every two years is valuable, with a pelvic examination at the same time, and that every year or two it is worthwhile checking the blood pressure, especially when machines to do it for fifty cents are rapidly becoming available in all the supermarkets. In the absence of any symptoms those provide the only significant benefits to be derived from costly physical examinations. It is prompt action when symptoms appear, rather than frequent examinations, that give you your best protection against death or disability.

Laboratory Tests

Since there are hundreds, if not thousands, of laboratory tests, it is obvious that most of them must be reserved for patients having symptoms that point to a specific disease and therefore call for a specific group of tests. There are, however, batteries of twelve or eighteen *sequential multiple analyses,* automated and therefore reasonably priced, called SMA-12 or SMA-18 depending on the number of tests done. These include testing the level of blood sugar to see if there is a tendency to diabetes, testing for kidney function, liver function, and function of the parathyroid glands. Sometimes the presence of cancers in bone also can be detected by these tests.

The trouble is that most of the blood tests find diseases for which there are no cures. These include diabetes, kidney

Annual Checkup and the Diagnosis of Surgical Problems

failure, or liver failure. Since we can't cure any of these diseases there is no advantage in discovering them early, before there are any symptoms. Probably it also is true that high calcium caused by overactivity of the parathyroid can be treated as satisfactorily after it causes symptoms as before, but because of the possibility that long exposure to high levels of calcium might damage the arteries and also because there may be *some* limited value in detecting and treating diabetes early, the SMA test should be done in people over forty once every three or four years. In the presence of symptoms, of course, the tests should be done at once.

Blood counts, to see if there is anemia or any abnormality in the number of white cells, are also done in the course of a routine survey. If there is anemia it is worth knowing about it, because occasionally it can indicate the presence of a still operable cancer of stomach or bowel. White blood cells also are counted, but if there are no symptoms, there is no particular value in finding out early that, for example, leukemia is present. It is no more curable early than late. The one blood test that is of value is the test for syphilis. Over a period of ten years or so, undetected syphilis can cause irreversible damage to the nervous system. For this reason sexually active people should be tested for syphilis every five or ten years, even if there are no symptoms of the disease.

From the foregoing, it is apparent that the chief responsibility for good health lies not with the physician who performs routine examinations and tests, nor with industries, insurance companies, or governments that sometimes subsidize periodic examinations, but with the patient himself, whose responsibility it is to keep watch over his own body and to report to his physician any changes or any symptoms. Enormous savings in health care could be made without sacrifice of longevity or comfort if people would become more responsible for their own welfare.

PART TWO

Surgical Care and Our Medical System

VI

Fee-for-Service Surgery

Why Doctors Don't Agree About Treatment

Many diseases are not scientifically understandable. For them, treatment must be empirical, based on observed results, rather than on proven theories. Different physicians, having had different experiences, will have observed different results. On the basis of these differences they will hold different opinions about treatment.

As an illustration of differences in experience resulting in different conclusions let us revert to one of the most common illustrations, the controversy about the treatment of cancer of the breast. If a surgeon has always treated cancer of the breast by radical mastectomy, he will never have seen good results following any other kind of surgical treatment. This is simply because the patients treated by simpler operations

Surgical Care
and Our Medical System

who are cured by them will have no need to consult a surgeon who prefers radical operations. All that surgeon will see, therefore, are the patients on whom simpler operations have failed. He will, therefore, conclude that simpler operations always fail. On the other hand, the surgeon who never does a radical operation will rarely be consulted by patients who are cured by radical operations. All he will see are patients with disasterous recurrences or side effects following radical surgery. This confirms his belief that the radical operation should never be done.

Another reason for differences of opinion among surgeons is differences in their patients. In many diseases, like gallstones, or nodules in the thyroid, the survival of the patient and the side effects of treatment depend on a number of factors, including the severity of the symptoms and the age and well-being of the patient. It is, therefore, impossible to generalize and say that this or that is the best treatment. The question is, "What is the best treatment for this particular patient?" By the same token, differences in skill among surgeons lead to differences of opinion as to whether or not an operation entails unacceptable risk.

As we have seen in earlier chapters, controversies in surgery rarely involve true differences in survival. In most cancers, for instance, survival depends not on how extensive the local treatment is but on whether or not the cancer has spread through the system before local treatment is given. There are many effective ways of treating the local cancer—by simple or radical operations, by extensive or localized radiation, by electrocoagulation (heat), or by cryotherapy (freezing). Any of these can destroy the local cancer, but none of them can cure the disease if it has already spread to distant parts of the body. That is why, so long as the local cancer is destroyed, there is little or no difference in survival regardless of the method of treatment. Controversy between

Fee-for-Service Surgery

doctors, therefore, generally revolves around side effects, complications, and discomforts of treatment.

A Built-in Conflict of Interest

Although the above considerations provide the basis for most of the disagreements about the best methods of treatment, there are other contributing factors. Training, practice, and economic pressures can push the surgeon's thinking in the direction of more frequent, more radical, and more remunerative surgery. It is not that the surgeon consciously decides to do an operation for economic reasons. The decision is more subtle, and is based on training and on habits of practice which through the years have been influenced by economic pressures, always in the same direction. If there is a question between operating or not operating, it is economically sound to operate. If it is a question of a big operation or a little one, it is better economy to do the big one. If it is a question of surgery versus radiation, it is surgery that gives the advantage to the surgeon. Finally, if it is a question of doing the operation oneself or referring the patient to a better-qualified specialist, it is obvious that there is little profit to be derived from referral.

At the heart of this trouble is our fee-for-service system. I believe that all hospital-based physicians, including surgeons and radiologists, should be paid salaries by hospitals instead of fees-for-service by their patients, by their insurers, or by Medicare or Medicaid. This method would tend to decrease the present conflicts of interest.

"As to the honor and conscience of doctors, they have as much as any other class of men, no more and no less. And what other men dare pretend to be impartial where they

Surgical Care and Our Medical System

have a strong pecuniary interest on one side?" George Bernard Shaw wrote these lines in his Preface to *The Doctor's Dilemma*. He concludes that "it is simply unscientific to allege or believe that doctors do not under existing circumstances perform unnecessary operations and manufacture and prolong lucrative illnesses."

Today in the United States "existing circumstances" are similar to those that Shaw was writing about in England in 1911—namely, fee-for-service surgery in which the surgeon is paid according to whether he decides to operate and according to the extent, danger, and complexity of the operation that he selects. Why is the United States the only advanced western country in which fee-for-service surgery persists as the usual form of payment? There is indeed only one profession in which conflict of interest is not only tolerated but even extolled as a shining example of the free-enterprise system. That is medicine, and particularly surgery.

The Effect of Conflict of Interest

Conflict of interest occurs when a person who is acting as a judge has personal interests that are affected by the decision. Thus the surgeon who decides whether or not he should perform an operation is faced with a conflict of interest; he is paid if he operates and he isn't paid if he doesn't. The surgeon faces a further conflict of interest if he has a choice between performing a major operation for a large fee or a minor one for which the fee might be only a fifth as much. Finally, if he knows that he is not expert at a certain type of operation that others could perform better and more safely, his decision whether to perform the operation himself or to

Fee-for-Service Surgery

call in a specialist is again subject to a conflict of interest. In short, there are many surgical decisions in which the best interest of the patient is in sharp conflict with the financial interest of the surgeon. Since in such cases the surgeon is the judge, we are reminded of Shaw's statement that a judge whose pay "depended on whether the verdict was for plaintiff or defendant . . . would be as little trusted as a general in the pay of the enemy."

The conflict of interest presented to the surgeon is not to the patient's advantage. When there is a question of whether an operation is needed or not, the patient usually is happier if the decision is not to operate. Yet the surgeon making this decision stands to earn a fee of $500 if he decides to operate and nothing at all if he decides not to.

Although I do not believe that surgeons are consciously influenced by the consideration of the possible fee, I am sure that over a period of years, the financial pressure, always exerted in the same direction, tends to make surgeons rationalize their decisions, look for excuses to operate instead of for reasons not to, and results in their teaching their successors the same rationalizations and the same excuses for doing ever more surgery.

The American system negates the results of scientific research, subjects our citizens to increased suffering and risks of death, and is one of the reasons why in the past fifty years, in spite of all the so-called advances in surgery and medicine, the average life expectancy of a man at fifty has increased by only a few months.

Industrialists work for salaries. So do judges, and so do the surgeons in the armed forces, the Veterans' Administration, almost all of the large clinics, and many of the universities. There is really nothing novel about the idea of having surgeons paid by salary. Moreover, it makes the surgeon a part of a cooperating health team instead of an individualistic

SURGICAL CARE
AND OUR MEDICAL SYSTEM

entrepreneur. What is being advocated is not socialized medicine. It is rather the same type of private enterprise and specialization that has produced the triumphs of American productivity, substituting organized factories for a scattered cottage industry. As a compromise between the present unsatisfactory system of fee-for-service medicine and a system of state medicine (which, no matter how organized, would be apt to be a disaster), I am urging that hospital-based specialists, including surgeons, anesthesiologists, pathologists, oncologists, cardiac catheterization specialists, and any other type of physician whose practice is based in the hospital rather than in his office, be paid by the hospital rather than directly by the patient. The fees for the services of these physicians would be collected by the hospital—a nonprofit institution, of course—and would be used to pay the salaries of the physicians and to support the facilities of the hospital or to lower the fees and reduce the cost of medical care.

Effect of the Method of Remuneration on the Number of Operations Done

Dr. C. B. Esselstyn, Sr., has reported that among the members of a prepaid health plan staffed by salaried physicians, the incidence of major surgical operations was 33 per 1,000 compared to 69 per 1,000 in a similar group of people that elected to be cared for on a fee-for-service basis.[1] In the prepayment plan the patient paid a certain sum each year and it was the Plan's responsibility to take care of all of the patient's illnesses without further charge. It was, therefore, to the financial interest of the Plan to avoid unnecessary operations. In the fee-for-service, Blue-Shield type of plan,

Fee-for-Service Surgery

on the other hand, the surgeon who made the decision whether to operate was paid a fee if he operated and was not paid if he didn't. It is hard to avoid the conclusion that this arrangement had something to do with the fact that twice as many operations were done on the fee-for-service patients.

Dr. Esselstyn went on to discuss the traditional fee-for-service basis of medical care, calling it the "piecework" basis for medical care: "The principle of piecework," he said, "was invented as an incentive to encourage the production of more pieces. Over the years it has been found to be effective not only in certain industries but in medical care as well."

In a January 8, 1973 article in *Medical Economics* entitled "What Makes Americans So Operation-Happy," it was reported that "Americans have operations at double the British rate."[2] "I know of a case," said Dr. Ken L. White of Johns Hopkins in the same article, "when a physician was making a helluva lot of money performing tonsillectomies on a fee-for-service basis. Then he went on an annual retainer and his tonsillectomy rate dropped sharply. He was just as startled as anyone else; he hadn't been consciously pushing tonsillectomies, just performing them routinely."

The same article cited another interesting study by Dr. J. P. Bunker of Stamford, who compared operations done in the United States with those done in England and Wales. He, too, found that twice as many operations per capita were performed in the United States and related this to the fact that in this country there were twice as many surgeons per capita. Doctor Bunker concluded that the method of payment appeared to play an important if unmeasured part, and that the incentive of fee-for-service may tend to increase the number of operations in cases in which indications are borderline. These figures should not be taken to mean that more operations insure better health. Other studies, for example, have shown that the overall mortality rate from appendicitis, including the deaths that occurred from appendectomy, were highest in the areas with the most operations for appendicitis.[3]

Effect of the Size of Fee on the Operation Selected

My own experience in trying to change what I have considered to be outdated surgical practices has been chiefly in the field of thyroid and breast disease. My efforts have been directed toward simplifying treatment, taking advantage of modern advances in diagnosis to avoid unnecessary operations, and substituting simple operations for radical ones. From the economic standpoint, however, such changes reduce income. In a fee-for-service system the more the surgeon operates, and the bigger the operations he does, the better off he is. I will give some examples. One insurance carrier does not wish to have its fee schedule published in terms of dollars, but gave me the following information about the relative fees for different operations. Valuing the largest general-surgical operations such as resection of the rectum at 100, various operations on the breast were valued as follows:

Radical mastectomy	75
Modified radical mastectomy	55
Simple mastectomy	45
Partial mastectomy	25
Open biopsy	15
Needle biopsy	8

Fee-for-Service Surgery

(The last item refers to a complicated in-hospital biopsy. On the same scale, needle aspiration of a breast cyst or aspiration biopsy of a tumor in the office would rate 1.5 to 2.5.)

Not all physicians agree that the size of payment affects decisions about treatment. When, in a newspaper interview, I suggested that the fact that the insurance carriers paid surgeons more for big operations than for small ones might have something to do with the continuing popularity of radical mastectomy, there was a sharp reaction from the local medical community. The Ethics Committee of the Cleveland Academy of Medicine (American Medical Association) asked me to appear, and then, disregarding the fate of the 90,000 new women who each year will be treated for breast cancer, the committee concluded that I should not have informed the press of my belief that radical mastectomy was archaic and no longer necessary. It made surgeons who had treated patients by radical operations "subject to criticism by their patients," the committee explained.

Surgical decisions would be clear and easy if medical science had progressed to the point that all agreed which treatment was best. Since this utopia is not yet here, economic considerations sometimes motivate the physician to accept that part of the scientific evidence that best supports the method that gives him the most money. An example discussed in Chapter II is the use of the needle as an inexpensive office procedure, to aspirate the contents of a cyst of the breast. Dr. George Rosemond, President of the American Cancer Society, has written eloquently on this subject,[4] urging surgeons to treat cysts in the office by simple aspiration. Yet there are areas in the country where most surgeons admit their patients to the hospital and remove the cysts and surrounding tissue, expounding to their patients the long-since-disproved theory that this avoids any danger of spreading the tumor in case it is malignant. Replies to a question-

Surgical Care and Our Medical System

naire sent by a medical school to surgeons of New Jersey, for example, showed that 42 percent of them never used a needle for aspiration and 27 percent of them rarely did. Is it possible that these findings are related to the fact that the aspiration of a cyst in the office commands such a small fee as compared to that obtained by an open operation?

Human nature is much the same throughout the world. On a recent trip to Spain I met a surgeon who worked in one of the Spanish Social Security hospitals. In the course of our discussion I asked him what operation was commonly used to treat breast cancer. "Simple or modified mastectomy in the Social Security Hospitals," he replied, "but most surgeons do the radical mastectomy on the private patients that they treat in their clinics." The latter, of course, paid their surgeons by fee-for-service, and the bigger the service the bigger the fee.

Referrals

A surgeon's practice consists largely of patients referred to him by other physicians. In order to have a constant stream of referrals, the surgeon must please the referring physicians. Sometimes this is best accomplished by doing what those physicians approve of or want done. When these desires run contrary to the best judgment of the surgeon, conflicts of interest again appear. If the surgeon does what he thinks his colleagues expect, he may not be doing what he believes is in the best interests of his patient.

I do not mean to imply that the referring physician is often in conflict with the surgeon. Moreover, the physician's judgment may be right and the surgeon's wrong. Nevertheless, some physicians become accustomed to dic-

Fee-for-Service Surgery

tating both diagnoses and treatments, and expect the specialists to comply. It is then that conflicts of interest arise. A friend of mine, an elderly internist, had had intermittent abdominal pain for some years. Finally, he had a typical attack of acute appendicitis. The appendix was removed, and thereafter the internist had little or no abdominal pain. Thereafter, also, he advised appendectomy for any patient with vague abdominal pain, a procedure that rarely relieved the symptoms and, of course, resulted in the needless removal of many normal appendices. The internist knew that none of the mature and experienced surgeons of the staff would go along with his diagnoses and suggestions for treatment. Invariably, therefore, he referred the patient to the youngest upstart on the surgical staff, always with a telephone call or note indicating clearly what he thought was wrong and that appendectomy was the treatment. Flattered to have a case referred personally by the senior internist and afraid of offending him by not complying, many of the young surgeons would go ahead and remove these appendices. Their willingness to comply was now established and their practices were enhanced by a steady stream of patients referred for unwarranted appendectomies.

In the last twenty years, surgery has become more complex and more specialized. Not only has the general surgeon stopped dabbling in such specialties as neurosurgery, orthopedics, and urology, but the gynecologists have largely taken over the pelvis, and the thoracic surgeons, the chest. Vascular surgeons often do most of the blood-vessel surgery, and more and more of the plastic surgery and the specialized surgery of the colon and rectum is going to specialists in these fields. Even within what is left of general surgery there is specialization, some surgeons limiting their practice to the surgery of children, others to the treatment of cancer, others

SURGICAL CARE AND OUR MEDICAL SYSTEM

having special interests in surgery of the thyroid, parathyroid, pancreas, breast, etc.

Usually the surgeon who has a special field of interest will have more experience in this field than his more generalized colleagues, and as a result of this experience his competence increases. This gives rise to a conflict of interest for the general surgeon. If a patient requires a relatively rare and complicated operation which the general surgeon does not often do, the surgeon must decide whether or not to refer the patient to a specialist who would perform the operation better and with less risk than himself. If he decides to do the operation himself he gets paid; if he refers the patient to a specialist he does not.

I do not imply that the need to make this decision arises often, for most operations—hysterectomy, appendectomy, removal of the gallbladder, repair of a hernia—are not only common but are not particularly dangerous or complicated. Probably they are performed about as safely and as well by any qualified and experienced general surgeon as by a surgeon with a special interest. But in more extensive, uncommon, and dangerous operations, as we have seen in Part One, the chances of survival are closely related to the judgment, skill, and experience of the surgeon. In these the risk of operation varies by a ratio of as much as 10 to 1, depending on who does it.

Unfortunately, the cards are stacked against the patient. If the surgeon decides to do a big operation himself he may collect a minimum fee of $1,000. If he refers the patient to a specialist he receives a $25 consultation fee. In all of the decision-making process the patient has little to say. He does not know or ask about the surgeon's training, experience, or mortality rate. Nor is the surgeon apt to volunteer this information. That is why I believe that hospital mortality rates should be published as a means of allowing the patient to

Fee-for-Service
Surgery

know what risk he is running and of helping to give him that most important of his rights, informed consent. It is worth traveling to a specialized center if safe, high-quality treatment is not available at home.

The Role of the Hospital

One of the disturbing features of medical practice is the profession's inability to deal with its own shortcomings. For example, there was a surgeon on the staff of a community hospital near Cleveland who was notorious in medical circles for performing unnecessary operations. The leading surgeons of the staff met together and appointed delegates to present the evidence to the board of trustees and to ask them to suspend the surgeon's operating privileges. The trustees complied. The surgeon sued the hospital, the trustees, and the other surgeons individually and collectively for millions of dollars. Had the case come to court it would have taken hundreds of man-hours of work on the part of the surgeons to assemble and present the evidence. The surgeon was reinstated and the case was dropped.

Had the surgeon who was suspended been employed by the hospital and remunerated by a salary, it is unlikely that he would have been tempted to perform unnecessary operations. If through poor training or bad judgment he did a large number of unnecessary operations, or if he consistently had poor results due to faulty judgment or technique, his services could have been terminated. But as a member of the visiting staff, practicing fee-for-service medicine, he could not be suspended without being proven to be at fault.

The conflicts of interest and the temptations built into fee-for-service surgery are less marked in the large private

Surgical Care and Our Medical System

clinics, most of which are incorporated not for profit and practically all of which pay their physicians by salary. The salary may be related to the number of operations done by the individual, but it is based also on quality of work, research, teaching, and executive ability of the individual. In short, although there is still incentive to generate a professional income, all money collected for professional services goes to the institution. Already the surgical departments of several medical schools have adopted this type of system, and a number of community hospitals have begun to put the chief of the service on full salary, making him responsible for teaching and for the organization of the service. I see no reason why, gradually over the next twenty years, the entire surgical staff of most hospitals should not be similarly organized.

Most established surgeons are too set in their habits of practice to make a sudden change. It is on the habits of practice of the young surgeon, struggling to make a living, that the change would have its greatest effect. Therefore, I think that the effect of a change in the system of paying for operations would be delayed for nearly half a generation until the young surgeons who started out by being paid a straight salary came to maturity and began to perform most of the nation's operations. At that time I believe the quality of surgery would be vastly improved.

In the meantime, even before the fee-for-service system of surgical practice is changed to one in which the surgeon is paid by salary, it would be helpful if the hospitals in which the surgeons worked took more care to see that their mortality rates were acceptably low. This they could easily accomplish by refusing to let unqualified and unspecialized surgeons perform the more complex and hazardous operations.

VII

Surgery Under State Medicine, Prepaid Health Plans (HMO), and Fee-for-Service

In the United States, most health care is given by private practitioners, whereas in socialist countries, it is given by salaried employees of the state. There are fundamental differences between these two types of health care, and also between these and the type of care that is given under prepaid health maintenance plans, like the Kaiser Foundation's. These differences can affect both the frequency and nature of surgery and its cost. The situation can be summarized as follows:

1. In *fee-for-service private practice,* the more thoroughly the patient is studied and the more extensively he is treated, the more money the physician makes. This may lead to the best possible diagnosis and treatment or

Surgical Care and Our Medical System

it may result in abuses, such as overdiagnosis and overtreatment, including surgery, and in the exploitation of Medicare and insurance funds. In fee-for-service private practice, however, there is one bonus that both the private physician and his patient can get, and that is a warm and satisfactory personal relationship. A further benefit for the patient is the choice of physician, or the chance to shop around for the most highly qualified surgeon.

2. Under *prepayment plans,* such as that of the Kaiser Foundation or similar health maintenance organizations (HMO), the patient pays in advance for a specified period of medical care. Since the payment is no more for much service than for little, the less that is done in the way of tests, treatments, and hospitalization, the less will be the cost to the organization and the more money it will make. However, if the organization is incorporated as not for profit, as in the case with Kaiser, there is no reason for it to put pressure on its physicians to undertreat their patients. If a patient were undertreated, it would be because it is less work for the doctor to undertreat. His salary is the same. Under prepayment plans, although the patient may have some choice of physician, it is only within the staff of the organization.

3. In a *socialized practice,* like England's, funded by the state, there is likewise no economic incentive to overtreat. Since the general practitioner is paid on a capitation basis, according to the number of patients that are on his panel, there may be a temptation to accept more patients than he can serve satisfactorily. This, as in the HMO prepayment plan, could result in undertreatment. It is also easier for the general physician to refer his

Surgery Under State Medicine, Prepaid Health Plans (HMO), and Fee-for-Service

time-consuming problems to a hospital-based specialist. But, in the impersonality of the government's footing the bill, there is no incentive to keep patients out of the hospital or for the salaried, hospital-based specialists to keep down their patients' in-hospital expense or length of stay.

I have practiced medicine mainly in the Cleveland Clinic, which is a sort of hybrid between fee-for-service private practice and socialized medicine. This has given me some insight into the problems of both. The large clinics like Mayo, Cleveland, Ochsner, and Lahey take from private practice the necessity of pleasing the patient and of charging him a reasonable fee. They take from socialized practice the custom of paying the physician a salary. The hybrid clinic corporation practices fee-for-service medicine, but the individuals within it are socialized to such a degree that their value to the institutional organism depends as much on their willingness to cooperate as on the dollars they earn individually in their various specialties.

I cannot see why a well-motivated, highly qualified physician or surgeon would be any less effective in a socialized than in a private setting. This deduction is based on the observations of socialized hospital practice that I have seen in Russia, Europe, Japan, Greece, Thailand, Hong Kong, Taiwan, Bali, and Fiji, as well as in the United States Navy in World War II. In India and Haiti, where socialized medicine and private practice may coexist, I saw excellent surgical technique, usually learned abroad, but sometimes there were appalling priorities. In Bombay, for instance, the chief of surgery had just retreated to his sumptuous, air-conditioned suite after doing two heart transplants, while his hospital was so crowded that there was a patient on the floor between each filled bed. And in Haiti, while children were

Surgical Care and Our Medical System

losing their fingers and toes from the ergotlike effect of Bush Tea and scores of babies were dying of diarrhea, the American-trained surgical chief had scheduled an adrenalectomy on an octogenarian with breast cancer and a repair of a painless aortic aneurysm in a man of seventy-five. In America, too, I have seen exploitation in the form of overtreatment. It is this and the overuse of hospitals and of diagnostic tests that, in my opinion, are going to lead to the socialization of American medicine.

At first the socialization may be on a fee-for-service basis, a Medicare type of "let the government pay" plan. But when the bills start coming in, this will change. The government will not be able to afford the abuses of fee-for-service. Eventually physicians and surgeons will be paid by salary, and the salary won't be higher than that of the politician who sets it.

But there are other possibilities. I think we must consider the government's efforts to multiply and enlarge the Kaiser-like prepayment schemes, or HMO's, that offer the most effective way to cut the cost of medical care. In a prepayment scheme, there is no incentive to overtreat. The danger is that, without incentive or competition, the treatment will be inadequate. On the other hand, if all the medical services of the country were delivered by private practitioners, or even by private, fee-for-service clinics, there would be no escape from the incentives to overtreat, or perform inappropriate or too-elaborate surgery.

I can think of no compromise between the prepayment and the fee-for-service systems. The answer may be to let them compete so that dissatisfied patients can go from one system to the other. Competition would tend to lower the cost of fee-for-service medicine and to raise the quality and dignity of prepaid care.

I do not believe that the government can practice medicine as effectively as competitive nonfederal corporations.

Surgery Under State Medicine, Prepaid Health Plans (HMO), and Fee-for-Service

For example, the Washington *Star*, in September 1977, reported that a study made by a House Investigations subcommittee showed that patients eligible for Medicaid had "twice the rate of surgery for the United States as a whole." The current cost to the federal government of Medicaid was given as $7 billion a year. My opinion, therefore, is that we should work to develop the prepayment plans until they constitute 50 percent of the country's medical practice. Then we should try to save the fee-for-service practitioners and clinics, which by that time will be in considerable financial trouble. When we have attained these ends, medicine will have a two-party system, like the Republicans and Democrats!

VIII

Inappropriate Operations and How to Eliminate Them

Functionlust

The foregoing chapter implies that if surgeons were paid straight salaries all conflicts of interest would cease and that a new era would dawn. Unfortuantely, it is not as simple as that. The temptation of fee-for-service is only one of the factors involved in decision-making. The others are more subtle and more difficult to control. I refer to professional pride and to what might be called, in the term of Konrad Lorenz, *functionlust*.

Surgery combines science, art, and skill. The judgment of a surgeon is based mainly on his mastery of science. The art of surgery depends on adapting the operation to the needs of the particular patient. The skill of the surgeon is based on

Inappropriate Operations
and How to Eliminate Them

his innate technical ability supplemented by his training and experience.

The gifted surgeon who operates rapidly, carefully, and with consummate skill is justly proud of his ability. He enjoys operating just as a ballet dancer enjoys dancing or a skilled weaver enjoys weaving. This is functionlust—the love of doing a thing, and functionlust can be a temptation to surgeons and can provide almost as sharp a conflict of interest as fee-for-service.

A surgeon may be highly skilled in some fields of surgery, that of the colon for example, but may have never learned to do any operation for cancer of the rectum except the radical resection with colostomy. This he does routinely for all rectal cancers, justifying the procedure by the unwarranted conclusion that because this operation is the biggest it is necessarily the best. Specialists in this field could save the rectum and avoid colostomy in many cases, but performing the radical operation that this surgeon does so quickly, so skillfully, and so safely is such a source of satisfaction to him that his mind precludes investigation of the other methods. The same may be true in the case of surgeons who have learned to be expert in performing the radical mastectomy for breast cancer. Functionlust provides a temptation that makes it hard to accept changes in the scientific data on which the use of his operation is based. "My results are good," the surgeon says. "Why change?" So he continues to perform his favorite operation.

SURGICAL CARE
AND OUR MEDICAL SYSTEM

Inappropriate Operations

We have seen that there are a number of large, deforming, or dangerous operations that in many cases can be supplanted by less radical and less dangerous operations without diminishing the chances of cure. There are also a number of diseases that can be treated equally effectively by methods other than surgery. Finally, there are a number of operations that used to be done commonly but which now are considered to be unnecessary. Among these is suspension of the uterus for retroversion (a bent-backward position of the organ that some years ago was thought to be a common cause of backache). Another is tonsillectomy, which fifty years ago was considered almost mandatory for the good health of a child. (My father was a surgeon, and all four of his children had their tonsils out.) Appendectomy was also in high vogue, the fear of appendicitis being so great that patients requested and physicians often advised appendectomy merely to prevent the possibility of getting appendicitis. (This happened to one of my sisters.) In those days no one accused surgeons of doing unnecessary operations, yet their most common operations are now deemed unnecessary or inappropriate.

The foregoing historical examples of inappropriate operations, widely done by distinguished and respected surgeons, makes it appear likely that the inappropriate operations done today are done for the same reasons as in the past—not because of a conscious desire for profit but because of the traditions of the profession and the way surgeons are taught. To do these inappropriate operations is a style of practice.

When the fee-for-service system of surgery makes it highly profitable to perform as many and as large operations as possible, and when Blue Shield insurance pays much more for the large, dangerous, and disabling operations than for

Inappropriate Operations
and How to Eliminate Them

conservative ones, there is little incentive for the surgeon to change his ways. In 1976 the *Bulletin of the American College of Surgeons* stated that "The Federal Employees Program under Blue Cross and Blue Shield auspices listed nearly half a million dollars in payments for the presumably abandoned operation of sympathectomy for hypertension and more than half that amount for uterine suspension procedures. Payments for other outmoded operations contribute further to the waste of our limited resources, as does the wanton use of new diagnostic tests without omitting the tests they are designed to replace."[1] The *Bulletin* goes on to say that the decision appears to lie between surgeons changing their ways so as to lower expenses, or accepting Federal intervention.

The *Bulletin* does not mention the other alternative, which I think would solve the problem. That is abolishing fee-for-service surgery and substituting payment by salaries from hospitals. The hospitals in turn would be required to make available to inspection the number of each type of operation that was done so that a central inspection group could decide if too many obsolete or inappropriate operations were being done. Some sort of change is essential, because unless the medical profession reforms itself there are forces at work that may well drive this country into completely socialized medicine. This could soon result in a bitter and discontented medical profession and in a less than satisfactory relationship between physicians and patients. In the meantime, it would be helpful if the public knew more about what operations are unnecessary or inappropriate.

SURGICAL CARE
AND OUR MEDICAL SYSTEM

Recognizing Inappropriate Operations

During 1976, in congressional committees and in a series of articles in *The New York Times*, there was much discussion of unnecessary operations. The American Medical Association in turn challenged the charges that an excessive number of unnecessary operations are performed. Unfortunately, there is no way to resolve this debate, because there is no way to define a "necessary" operation. What is it necessary for? For survival? For comfort? For safety? For birth control? For beauty? Or, as in circumcision, for tradition? It would be simpler if we stopped using the terms *necessary* and *unnecessary* and substituted *appropriate* and *inappropriate*. There are three types of inappropriate operations.

1. Operations in which surgery is not an appropriate treatment for the disease. This may be because there is no disease, as is the case with most tonsillectomies, or it could be because the disease could be controlled as effectively by no treatment or by medical treatment. For example, a forty-eight-year-old woman has a small fibroid of the uterus which is giving no symptoms and whose presence entails no risk. No treatment is needed, because after the menopause the fibroid will shrink or disappear. However, if the physician mentions tumors of the uterus without explaining, the woman may believe she has a cancer and accept the unnecessary risk of operation.

A forty-five-year-old woman has a hard, round lump in the breast. It is a typical cyst, but instead of aspirating the fluid, a treatment that cures 99 percent of breast cysts, the surgeon admits the patient to the hospital and, with signed consent for a mastectomy if

Inappropriate Operations
and How to Eliminate Them

necessary, subjects her to the expense of complete preoperative studies, anesthesia, and of an operation to remove the cyst.

There are inflammations of the thyroid, known as *thyroiditis,* which respond specifically to medical treatment, the goiter shrinking or disappearing. The diagnosis can be confirmed easily by needle biopsy done in the office. Nevertheless, every year thousands of operations (thyroidectomies) are done, inappropriately, for thyroiditis.

2. An operation, or the type of operation chosen, was not appropriate for the individual. A seventy-year-old overweight woman has gallstones that were discovered accidentally on an x-ray taken for other reasons. The stones were causing no symptoms, a common situation in older people. Although it could be argued that in a healthy, young person removal of the gallbladder would be justified because the stones might eventually cause complications, the risk of operation on an overweight woman in her seventies would greatly outweigh the benefits to be derived from removing stones that were causing no symptoms. The operation would, therefore, be inappropriate for the individual patient.

An eighty-year-old man has a low-lying rectal cancer, for which the surgeon advises a radical resection of the rectum. At that age, the risk of the radical operation far outweighs any theoretical benefit of resection over local destruction of the cancer by heat or radiation.

A woman of fifty has hyperthyroidism typical of Graves' disease. Treatment by radioactive iodine is an accepted method of treatment. Although there is argument that the radiation may produce side effects in young people, there is no reason why in older people

Surgical Care and Our Medical System

radioactive iodine should not be used routinely in order to avoid the expense, discomfort, and risk of operation. To operate on such a patient would be inappropriate because of age.

3. Rare or dangerous operations may be inappropriate because the surgeon was not trained to perform the operation expertly. Common operations such as repair of a hernia or removal of the uterus or gallbladder are relatively safe and are apt to be done about as well in one hospital as in another. The opposite is true of some of the rare and dangerous operations. Here the mortality rates —that is to say, the chance of dying as a direct result of the operation—vary by a ratio of as much as 10 to 1. This is because the operations are not common; hence, unspecialized surgeons have not had enough experience in doing them to have developed a technique that is safe.

An example of the high mortality rates that sometimes occur when rare and difficult operations are done in unspecialized hospitals occurred in a community hospital in Massachusetts, where the mortality rate of open-heart surgery was 52 percent. This does not mean that there was a 52 percent chance of dying of the disease; it means there was a 52 percent chance of dying of the operation. This mortality is ten times as high as is generally expected and nearly twenty times as high as the best reported results. As noted earlier, there are similar differences in mortality rates following other dangerous operations, such as those for cancers of the pancreas and of the rectum. The lowest mortality rates are always in the hospitals where a surgeon or surgical group has made a specialty or subspecialty of that narrow branch of surgery.[2]

Inappropriate Operations and How to Eliminate Them

These are examples of operations that are inappropriate in each of the categories. What can be done to insure that they will not continue to be done? I believe the easiest way to accomplish this is to pass a law that would order hospitals to report both the mortality rates of standard operations and the number of each type of operation done.

Most hospitals have what is known as a tissue committee that reviews the tissues that are removed. If too high a proportion of normal appendices, gallbladders, or uteri are removed, the offending surgeons are apt to be reprimanded. If they persist they may lose their operating privileges. But this is rare, because the most common abuses do not involve removing normal tissues. That is why most operations cannot be recognized as unnecessary or even as inappropriate simply by determining whether or not the tissue removed was normal or abnormal. To know whether the operation was appropriate, it is necessary to know also what the mortality rates of the operations were and the proportion of each type done. This would be easy if each hospital were required to publish its mortality rates for all standard operations and also the number of operations of each type done, such as tonsillectomies and hysterectomies, and the number of breast cysts that were excised instead of being aspirated and the proportion of goiters that were removed for thyroiditis. The tissue diagnoses of the pathologists should also be recorded so that anyone reviewing the records could note an inordinately high proportion of normal appendices, tonsils, gallbladders, or uteri. All of these reports could be reviewed periodically by a committee from the American Medical Association, the American College of Surgeons, or the American Hospital Association.

If in any hospital mortality rates of standard operations were unduly high or if there were too many tonsils or normal uteri removed, the hospital could be investigated more

SURGICAL CARE
AND OUR MEDICAL SYSTEM

thoroughly. If it were determined that too high a proportion of the operations were inappropriate, the hospital could be warned that its records would be reinspected in a year. If the abuses were not corrected the hospital would lose its approval. This, in turn, would mean that patients whose expenses were paid by Medicare and Medicaid could no longer be admitted. Since few hospitals could survive such a blow, it is likely that the staffs of the hospitals would identify the surgeons who were doing inappropriate operations and see to it that those surgeons corrected their ways or stopped operating. In short, if reporting the results of operations were mandatory, the staffs of hospitals would have a strong incentive to correct abuses, a goal that would be difficult, if not impossible, for a federal agency to impose on the individual surgeons.

Informed
Consent

scientific studies, since well-qualified surgeons do not always agree, and since the patients of today are not only literate, but quite well acquainted with surgical problems, as presented in the women's magazines and news magazines, the time seems long overdue to involve the patient in surgical decision-making.

This would seem to be simple enough, but there is disagreement about the feasibility of obtaining informed consent. An editor who read this manuscript noted that informed consent was difficult, if not impossible, to achieve. "The doctor's knowledge is so much greater than the patient's," he said. "In decisions involving cancer," he explained, "the situation is even more difficult. The superstitious dread of cancer that some of us live with horribly distorts our relationship with our doctors. Moreover, cancer is only a metaphor of the way we view all disease, to the point that our bodies become, not vessels of life, but the hosts of an antilife called malignancy."

I believe there is much truth in the editor's words but that instead of negating the necessity for informed consent they give it strong support. It would be tragic to believe that in this day of universal literacy people cannot be educated to understand the basic facts about various diseases and their treatment. If we do not do so, we may find ourselves in a situation similar to the Spanish Inquisition and at the mercy of a new kind of high priest. In our concern to exorcise disease we may sacrifice not only the quality of our lives but, in some cases, even life itself. Nor must we ever forget that one of the reasons for the persistence of the Spanish Inquisition was that all of the property of the one who was burned reverted to the Church. Along this same line some modern philosopher has stated, "If you accept the 'science' of the day you get burned in this world instead of in the next."

X

Public Education About Health

Ten years from now the practice of medicine will be quite different from today's. We are standing at the end of an era in which the public—and that means the patient—believed that the individual physician knew all the answers. This was because, until recently, physicians were in rather complete agreement about the stylized answers that they gave. For example, twenty years ago there was no surgical treatment of heart disease. Everyone agreed that digitalis was good. But today, there is no agreement as to the effectiveness of coronary bypasses and many other types of heart surgery.

A decade ago radical surgery was the accepted treatment of most cancers. The mortality and mutilation of the operations was not questioned by either patient or surgeon. Today, with the advent of superlative radiation therapy, and with the growing realization of the role of the immune system in

Public Education About Health

controlling the tumors' growth, physicians are no longer sure of the role of radical surgery. Informed by the press and television, many patients are beginning to look for less mutilating alternatives.

Kidney failure is no longer a question of diet and diuretics. It has become a debate between advocates of dialysis and transplantation. So it goes. Except in infectious disease, mastered by the antibiotics, everything is uncertainty. And into this area, where the truth is still obscure, has stepped the lawyer with a host of malpractice suits. Today, the physician is sued if he does and sued if he doesn't.

Looking to the future, I see that the surgeons of America will be dealing with patients who will be progressively better informed about medical and surgical treatments. When the surgeon is frank and open there will be a minimum of misunderstanding. If, on the other hand, surgeons continue to act as though they had the God-given right to do to the patient what they think best, they and their patients will be cast into an adversary position. The time is past where the patient can be viewed either as teaching material, as an unwitting part of an experiment, or as a subject on whom a favorite treatment can be practiced. The patient will have to be viewed as a full partner in the process of making decisions.

About 8 percent of the country's gross national product now goes to health-care expenditures. The 8 percent now being spent on health care—in a dream of prolonging life—is close to the 10 percent or "tithe" of everyone's income that was extracted by the clergy in the period when the power of the church was at its peak. However, whenever the tax that was demanded to attain eternal life exceeded 10 percent there followed a revolution against the clergy, and the state took over. Today, in the cost of health care, we are seeing an analogy to the tithe.

The cost of health care has entered a period of diminishing

Surgical Care
and Our Medical System

returns. Care is becoming more and more expensive. But if antibiotics, public-health measures, and standard of living are taken into consideration, it is difficult to prove that medical and surgical treatments are prolonging any more lives than they did when they were simpler and cheaper.[1] That is why people will soon refuse to pay so much. When this revolution comes it probably will result in a takeover of medicine by the state.

Representative Tim Lee Carter of Kentucky, himself a physician, was quoted in the *AMA News* as saying, "Only recently have we recognized that we no longer have the option of unlimited spending for personal health services." The insurance companies, unions, employees, and taxpayers are protesting the amount of money that goes to health care. In this situation, writes R. W. Cheadle, an old idea has been revived. "Why not teach health care to the patient so that he does not waste time and money consulting physicians about minor ills and show him how to adopt a healthier life style. Then perhaps he will be able to stay out of hospitals and require less medical care."[2]

Unexpressed but implicit in this new line of reasoning is the growing realization that medicine can only do so much. Health may be maintained better through education than by providing more medical services. Cheadle believes that there will soon be a drive towards "concerted national health education," as was started by President Nixon when he appointed a President's Committee on Health Education. It would be appropriate, at this time, to change the name of HEW (Health, Education, and Welfare) to EHW—putting Education in the prime position.

Dr. W. M. Carlyon of the AMA agrees. "Health education is here—and it's going to expand," he emphasizes. "Patients will find answers. If physicians don't help them find the right ones they will fill the information gap with misinformation

Public Education About Health

gleaned from a variety of dubious sources." That is the central body of the AMA speaking. Not yet come around to this broad view are all of the local chapters of the AMA, the academies of medicine of the individual cities or areas. These sometimes try to withhold medical information from the public for fear that the patients' increased knowledge might make them critical of the treatments that their physicians had given them in the past.

For example, in December 1977, at a meeting of the Cleveland Rotary Club, I had spoken about the desirability of patients' knowing their choices in surgery and their alternatives. Dr. Edward Kilroy, President of the Academy of Medicine, strode to the podium, and his remarks were reported by the *Cleveland Press* as follows: " 'Your physician should make the decision,' Kilroy said, fending off attempts [by the chairman] to interrupt him. 'The patient doesn't have the background to understand all these detailed problems.' " These remarks "drew boos from the Cleveland Rotary audience." In the face of the U.S. government's offer to pay for a second opinion about elective operations for Medicare-Medicaid patients, it is strange that a spokesman for organized medicine should urge the public to accept blindly whatever treatment is advised by the first surgeon consulted.

Because of this type of reaction from the professional organizations, I hope that control of the efforts to educate the public about medicine will be taken out of the hands of the local medical associations and be put into those of the universities, the central body of the AMA, or the government. In any case, it is time for the "ethics" of medical education for the public to be redesigned so that it is the patient who is protected instead of the doctor. The situation is reminiscent of the famous exchange in Joseph Heller's *Catch-22.* Yossarian says to the doctor:

Surgical Care
and Our Medical System

"That's just what I'm trying to tell you, goddammit. I'm asking you to save my life."

"It's not my business to save lives," Doc Daneeka retorted sullenly.

"What is your business?"

"I don't know what my business is. All they ever told me was to uphold the ethics of my profession and never give testimony against another physician."

XI

The Law of Diminishing Returns

In the treatment of disease, as in any other biological and therefore inexact science, there are negative as well as positive values. In general, the result is decided by the law of diminishing returns. Simple, inexpensive, and safe tests, used sparingly, may point the way to simple, inexpensive, and safe treatments that promote comfort and prolong life. On the other hand, complicated, expensive, and sometimes hazardous tests pointing the way to complicated types of treatment may result in more death and damage than would have occurred if no attempt had been made to diagnose or treat. That is why frequent complete examinations and early radical treatments may not result in longer survival, but to contrary results.

The following anecdote involved one of my colleagues, an

Surgical Care and Our Medical System

internist who specialized in doing annual physical examinations on executives of companies.

The patient was a man in his late forties who had had no symptoms referrable to colon or rectum. However, part of the annual physical examination contracted for by his company was a proctoscopic examination. When this was done, a very small cancer of the rectum was found, and the internist advised consultation with a surgeon. At the time, the most skillful colorectal surgeon of the area was out of town for a few days. The patient was so panicky and felt such urgency that he had his operation done by an unspecialized general surgeon in a community hospital. He died five days later from complications of the operation.

"In patients who had no symptoms, that is the only cancer of the rectum or colon that I ever picked up on routine proctoscopic examination," my colleague said. "Look what happened."

If diagnosis is carried to extremes, if every nodule in the thyroid is recognized and removed, if every lumpy area of the breast is excised, if every older person's gallbladder is x-rayed and all of those that contain stones are removed, if biopsies are taken of all nodules of the prostate and if all the malignant ones are treated by radical prostatectomy, if the gastrointestinal tract from mouth to anus is x-rayed and looked into regularly with the finding of large numbers of polyps and an occasional cancer and if all of the findings are corrected by operations, if all nodules of the skin that might possibly be skin cancer are removed, if all these things are done in the name of health, three things are bound to happen: Doctors will be rich, patients will be poor, and more people will die as a result of complications of the diagnostic tests or treatments than would have been saved by them.

I am not alone in my belief that there has been overemphasis of both diagnosis and treatment. At the annual meeting of

The Law of
Diminishing Returns

the American College of Surgeons in November 1976, the president, Dr. George R. Dunlop, gave an address entitled "Medical Costs—Our Common Dilemma." Dr. Dunlop pointed out that "the most important problem facing surgery today is the escalation of medical costs.

"It is little wonder that labor leaders are pressing for an all-inclusive national insurance program," Dr. Dunlop said, and went on to point out that in 1975 General Motors spent more money on health-insurance premiums for its employees than it paid to U.S. Steel, its major supplier of metal. Business finds that its contributions to the health-insurance premiums of its employees is such a large part of production costs that it is threatening to price their products out of the market. "Can a profession linked only by its concern for the sick and injured, which traditionally has concerned itself with the quality and not with the cost of medical care, be expected to provide the necessary answers to a concerned public?" Dr. Dunlop asked.

One of the problems is that the physician receives only 20 percent of the health-care dollar, and that an ever-increasing part of that is going via malpractice insurance to the lawyers. The other 80 percent of the health-care dollar goes to the hospital. The medical profession, partly to defend itself against threats of suits but also partly because of lack of self-discipline, has a tendency to overuse hospital facilities, not only hospitalization but also the expensive x-ray and laboratory tests that contribute so much to the cost of medical care. Although some of the tests and x-ray techniques are improvements over the old ways and may lead to better treatment, it is possible that more lives could be lengthened if the money were spent in other ways—for example, by a program to discourage children from starting to smoke. That is because medical care has a limited impact on health. A study of 226 critically ill patients requiring intensive care at the

Surgical Care
and Our Medical System

Massachusetts General Hospital showed that only 12 percent recovered for a total cost of $3,232,647, an average cost of $119,727 per recovery.[1] "What percentage of our national resources," asked Dr. Dunlop, "should be spent on health?" For example, already the kidney-dialysis program is costing the Federal Government more than $1 billion a year. It is estimated that by the late 1980s it will be costing $3 billion a year for the treatment of only 50,000 patients. What if, as a result of further technical advances, the artifical heart becomes available at a cost estimated at $20 billion a year?[2]

Every year new equipment is invented, much of it costly, like the $750,000 total-body computerized x-ray scanner. There are scores, if not hundreds, of expensive and sometimes valuable blood tests, many of them radioactive immuno-assays of incredible sensitivity. In special cases some of them can be of great value, but if they are widely used in screening, the cost soon becomes prohibitive, as in the widely publicized Medicaid scandal in which the government was bilked of millions of dollars in payment for unnecessary tests.

Another factor that is rapidly increasing the cost of medicine is malpractice insurance. Originally, the principle of the patient being able to sue the physician for damages incurred from negligence was a sound one, designed to make the physician more careful and to protect the rights of the patient. But now this principle has been carried too far, so that it has become a heavy financial burden, not on the physician, but on the patient to whom the cost of the physicians' insurance is passed on. Why should our politicians be required to divest themselves of holdings that involve a conflict of interest while our lawyers share the settlement with their clients?

It is no accident that malpractice insurance in the United States costs a surgeon at least twenty times as much as it would cost his English counterpart. This is because in En-

The Law of
Diminishing Returns

gland the taking of a "contingency fee"—the sharing of the settlement with the plaintiff—is called barratry, an offense that is illegal and punishable by fine or imprisonment. There is thus no temptation for the English lawyer to file an ill-founded suit in hopes that he will share in a settlement made, not because the defendant had done anything wrong, but to save the insurance company the expense of a suit. If fee-for-service for surgeons and the contingency fee for lawyers could be outlawed, it would go a long way toward raising the standards and reducing the cost of surgical care.

The action that might do the most to increase the cost of medical care is to pass the type of legislation that would make the state responsible for paying the people's health bills. This would be the greatest bonanza for physicians, technicians, drug companies, hospitals, and malpractice lawyers that was ever conceived. There would be neither economic nor quality control on the amount of health care given or of the technology used in delivering it. The cost of health care, already $118.5 billion, would rise to even more astronomical figures.

Man has never grudged the amount of effort he is willing to devote to perfect his technology or to implement his dreams of perpetual life. We need only to turn to history for analogies.

In prehistoric times, the Egyptians undertook and completed the building of the pyramids. For centuries they devoted a large proportion of their gross national product to this construction. No one knows why these vast edifices were built, but it is widely believed that their construction was motivated by some idea of eternal life. Or were they built simply because architects and engineers had discovered how to build them?

In the days of Greece and later of Rome, vast palaces and temples were built of huge blocks and columns of granite and

Surgical Care
and Our Medical System

marble, often transported from quarries thousands of miles away. During this period a high proportion of the gross national product went into the construction of these ceremonial buildings. Witness the monumental ruins of Baalbek. Was it to the gods that these temples were erected or to the technological glory of the vast columns that supported them?

Between 1194 and 1240 in a tiny village in France, the Cathedral of Chartres was built. The stated purpose of the cathedral was to house the garment that Mary wore when she bore Jesus, but the cathedral was 440 feet long and 377 feet high. Similar cathedrals were built in the Middle Ages throughout Europe, the technology spreading from country to country like that, in modern times, of the atomic bomb.

On a tiny land mass, far off the coast of Chile, the natives, perhaps in want of anything better to do, learned to sculpt and move vast images—the stone heads of Easter Island, standing up to 36 feet tall, one 66 feet long, all of them carved from solid stone. Why were these images cut and erected? Was it to prolong or perpetuate life? Or was it because the artisans had discovered how to carve and move the stone?

In later times man has continued to allow the pursuit of technology to dominate his actions. One of the major efforts of the twentieth century was to explore space and put a man on the moon. Is there an analogy between this journey and the construction of the pyramids, the cathedrals, and the images of Easter Island? Is there a further analogy between this and the current and apparently endless trend to try to prolong life through the technology of dialysis, kidney transplant, heart transplant, heart-lung machines, membrane oxygenators, and machines to assist circulation and respiration, all of them housed in the temples to science that we call hospitals? Is it practical for every woman over thirty-five years of age to have an annual mammogram—x-ray of the

The Law of
Diminishing Returns

breast—at a cost of $40 to $100, and involving, in younger women, some danger of inducing cancer by exposure to radiation? Is it reasonable to let the cost of malpractice insurance in many surgical specialties rise to from $20,000 to $40,000 per surgeon per year? Do the voters, who are the patients, realize that the cost of malpractice insurance is passed on to them or to their medical insurers and that often the lawyers get most of the money? Is it good economy or even good sense to have five or ten hospitals in each city competing for open-heart surgery when most of them don't do enough operations to maintain the professional competence of their personnel? Is it logical to have ten or more radiation-therapy centers in each city instead of one or two big ones, as is the custom in England, where each center treats hundreds of patients a day and can therefore afford the best equipment and personnel? Is it sensible to have rare, high-risk operations—such as those for cancers of the pancreas or rectum, or those for heart disease—performed at small community hospitals where surgeons and staffs are not specialized, highly trained, or highly practiced? Is it efficient to have what SOSSUS, the investigating committee of the American College of Surgeons and the American Surgical Association, considers to be 30 percent too many surgeons? The result is that the average surgeon does too few operations to enable him to gain skill from experience. Is it logical, in the face of this excess of surgeons, to continue to let surgeons go into practice, as many of them as please, with the result that there is a further diminution of the number of operations that each one does?

If the government simply paid the people's medical bills, is there any way that the indefinite proliferation of medical technology could be controlled? Is there any way that the predations of the malpractice lawyer, sharing the settlements with his clients, could be controlled if the government

Surgical Care and Our Medical System

simply picked up the tab for the physicians' ever-increasing fees? Would there be any end to the increasingly costly practice of "defensive medicine," requiring unnecessary or marginally necessary x-rays and laboratory tests in fear of being found negligent?

I remember when Blue Cross first started; it was about the time of the Great Depression. Before Blue Cross, the tests one ordered depended not only on what might help in diagnosis but also on what the patient could afford. Soon we found that before ordering laboratory tests or x-rays we were beginning to ask our patients whether or not they were insured. If they were it was considered good medicine to order all relevant tests. But I don't think that the insured ones got any better diagnosis as a result of the extra tests that were ordered. The essential ones were done anyway.

Whether it be in tests or in treatment, it is a fact that in all medical practice there is a law of diminishing returns. For example, the first time that a middle-aged woman has a mammogram, she has about five times the chance of something being found than she has on subsequent x-rays done once a year. In spite of all the advances in surgery and radiotherapy that have occurred in the last thirty years, the age-adjusted incidence of death from breast cancer has not changed. Again, and in spite of all advances in diagnosis and treatment since the turn of the century, there has been little increase in the life span of a man who has reached the age of sixty-five. This is because cells are not immortal, brain cells cannot be replaced, and man will continue to die of the complications of old age. It has also been estimated that even if all the common causes of death were miraculously abolished, the average life expectancy of man would be extended by only ten years, and those years would not be very happy or productive.[3] With the exception of antibiotics, most forms of treatment do not cure disease, they merely make life more

The Law of Diminishing Returns

comfortable and sometimes lengthen it a little. Preventive medicine, such as vaccinations and the control of pollution or of poisons in food and water, add more years to life than all of the so-called Miracles of Modern Medicine.

The question arises whether it would not be better to put some limit on medical expenses. Would it not be a better investment to devote more money to educating children about health, to controlling the abuse of drugs, to abolishing handguns, to rehabilitating criminals, and to increasing the safety of traffic? It is these considerations that make me feel that the problems of health care are being oversimplified and that the public is being misled by promises that more money spent on health will increase the span of life. The problem is more complicated than it appears. Today it is not so much health care as health education that is needed. In China, through education, venereal disease and the use of drugs were summarily abolished, and with their passing, crimes of violence also disappeared. In a highly literate country like ours, with the world's best system of communication, is there any reason that we cannot duplicate China's success?

Perhaps it is time that we recognized the limitations as well as the triumphs of medical and surgical treatments. If we do not, we may find that our hospitals have attained the preposterous stature of the Pyramids, the ancient temples, the medieval cathedrals, and Easter Island's stone figures. By that time no one will be able to remember quite why the hospitals were built. There they will stand, as they do today, often the largest building in the community—monuments to man's dedication to immortalizing his own technology.

If a limit is ever set on the growth of hospitals and on the proportion of the gross national product that can be spent on health, that limitation is not apt to come from the medical profession itself. If operations are simplified or supplanted by other methods of treatment, it is unlikely that it will be the

SURGICAL CARE
AND OUR MEDICAL SYSTEM

surgeons of the country who will initiate the change. In the Middle Ages it certainly was not the clergy who set limits on the number or the size of the cathedrals or on the taxes imposed on the people to support the church. It seems unlikely that it will be the lawyers of our country who will set limits on the proportion of the malpractice settlement that goes to the attorney. Thus, it is not the physicians but the people, the patients, who can do more than anyone else to limit the amount of money that will be spent on health.

Satchel Paige once said, "Don't look back—something might be gaining on you." One thing is certain, and that is that from the time we are born, something is gaining on us. By the time we are threescore years and ten, it has caught up with most of us. From the standpoint of health it doesn't pay for us to look back too often; we might see it and be frightened to death. From the standpoint of economy we can't pay for looking back too often and still afford to eat. It's better to wait until we feel that little tap on our shoulder and then talk it over with whatever it is that has caught up with us. The best rule for all of us to follow is to investigate any new symptom.

While we are waiting for that tap on the shoulder, we might do well to follow the advice of John Knowles, M.D., president of the Rockefeller Foundation, who, in an article entitled "The Responsibility of the Individual," argues very forcefully for increased health education.[4] Each individual, he maintains, should "support vastly increased funding to develop the best possible integration of health education into the school system, stressing measures that the individual can take to preserve his own health and knowledge about environmental hazards."

If in grade school we started teaching children, in the language of science, that it is their own decisions about their style of life—about cigarettes, alcohol, diet, and drugs—that

The Law of Diminishing Returns

will determine their health and survival, and if we taught them also about the value to their health of keeping in touch with the ever-changing technologies and philosophies of medical and surgical practice, then, when the time came, each of those persons would be better able to enter into the decision as to what treatment would be best for him or her as an individual.

Remember this about surgery:
There are risks.
There are benefits.
There are choices.
There are alternatives.
It is your body.
It is your life.
The final decision is yours.

Notes

Foreword

1. R. L. Varco and J. P. Delaney, *Controversy in Surgery* (Philadelphia: W. B. Saunders, 1976).

PART ONE
Chapter II

1. *Breast Cancer: A Report to the Profession 1976,* Supplement of *Cancer* 39 (June 1977).

2. F. C. Wood, *Journal of the American Medical Association* 73:-764–66 (1919).

3. George Crile, Jr., *What Women Should Know About the Breast Cancer Controversy* (New York: MacMillan, 1973); Rose Kushner,

Notes

Breast Cancer (New York: Harcourt Brace Jovanovich, 1975); Rosamond Campion, *The Invisible Worm* (New York: Macmillan, 1972); and Oliver Cope, *The Breast* (Boston: Houghton-Mifflin, 1977).

4. *The following is a summary of ten randomized trials comparing the survival of breast-cancer patients after various types of operation:*

a. A. P. M. Forrest et al., "The Cardiff-St. Mary's Trial," *British Journal of Surgery* 61: 766–69 (1974).
Simple mastectomy and axillary biopsy (radiation if nodes were involved) vs. radical mastectomy (radiation if nodes were involved).
Number of patients: 243 (randomized).
Duration of followup: 1 to 7 years.
Conclusion: simple mastectomy with selective postoperative radiotherapy is a safe policy of treatment.

b. S. Kaae and H. Johansen, "Simple vs. radical mastectomy for primary breast cancer." *Prognostic Factors in Breast Cancer* (Tenovus Symposium, 1st, Cardiff, Wales, 1967), A. P. M. Forrest and P. B. Kunkler, eds. (Baltimore: Williams & Wilkins, 1968).
Superradical mastectomy vs. simple mastectomy and radiation.
Number of patients: 425 (randomized).
Duration of followup: 10 years.
Conclusion: no difference; 42% were free of recurrence in both groups.

c. D. Brinkley and J. L. Haybittle, "Treatment of stage-II carcinoma of the female breast." *Lancet* 2: 1086–1087 (1971).
Simple mastectomy and radiation vs. radical mastectomy and radiation.
Number of patients: 204 (randomized).
Duration of followup: 5 to 12 years.
Conclusion: no difference in survival. Trial concluded because of increased morbidity in radical group.

d. J. I. Burn, "Early breast cancer; the Hammersmith trial." *British Journal of Surgery* 61: 762–765 (1974).
Simple mastectomy and radiation vs. radical mastectomy and radiation.
Number of patients: 195 (randomized).
Duration of followup: 4 to 9 years.
Conclusion: no difference in survival or local recurrence.

e. T. Hamilton, A. O. Langlands and R. J. Prescott, "The treatment of operable cancer of the breast; a clinical trial in the South-East Region of Scotland Trial." *British Journal of Surgery* 61: 758–761 (1974).

NOTES

Radical mastectomy vs. simple mastectomy and radiation.
Number of patients: 394 (randomized).
Duration of followup: 5 years.
Conclusion: "There is no significant difference in survival."
    f. J. G. Murray, "Cancer research campaign breast study." *British Journal of Surgery* 61: 772–774 (1974).
Clinical stages I and II.
Simple mastectomy alone vs. simple mastectomy and radiation.
Four months after simple mastectomy persistent nodes could be treated.
Number of patients: 2,000 (randomized).
Duration of followup 4 years.
Conclusion: "A larger number of people die within 3 years or have distant metastases in the irradiated group than in the watch policy group."
    g. L. Wise, A. Y. Mason, and L. V. Ackerman, "Local excision and irradiation; an alternative method for the treatment of early mammary cancer." *Annals of Surgery* 174: 393–401 (1971).
Radical mastectomy with or without radiation vs. partial mastectomy with or without radiation.
Number of patients: 186 (retrospective match).
Duration of followup: 10 years.
Conclusion: no significant difference in survival.
    h. V. Peters, "Cutting the gordian knot in early breast cancer." *Annals of the Royal College of Physicians and Surgeons*, Canada, pp. 186–192 (1975).
Radical mastectomy and radiation vs. local excision and radiation.
Number of patients: 434 (retrospective match).
Duration of followup: 10 years.
Conclusion: no difference in survival.
    i. J. Hayward, "Conservative surgery in the treatment of early breast cancer." *British Journal of Surgery* 61: 770–771 (1974).
Radical mastectomy and irradiation vs. wide local excision and irradiation.
Number of patients: 370 (randomized).
Duration of followup: 5 to 10 years.
Conclusion: "Wide excision with conservation of the breast must be considered a safe alternative to mastectomy in the treatment of patients with clinical stage I breast cancer."
    j. G. Crile, Jr., "Results of conservative treatment of breast cancer at 10 and 15 years." *Annals of Surgery* 181: 26–30 (1975).
Partial mastectomy with or without irradiation vs. total mastectomy with or without axillary dissection and radiation.
Number of patients: 84 (retrospective match).

Notes

Duration of followup: 10 years.
Conclusion: conservative and radical operations give the same rate of survival at 10 and at 15 years.

5. Wainwright Tumor Clinic Association of Pennsylvania, *The Surgical Treatment of Breast Cancer in Pennsylvania 1968–1973.*

6. Cope, *loc. cit.*

7. B. Fisher et al., *Annals of Surgery* 172 (1970).

8. K. McPherson and M. S. Fox, in *Costs, Risks, and Benefits of Surgery*, John P. Bunker, Benjamin A. Barnes, and Frederick Masteller, eds. (New York: Oxford University Press, 1977).

9. B. Fisher, *loc. cit.*

Chapter III

1. R. L. Varco and J. P. Delaney, *Controversy in Surgery* (Philadelphia: W. B. Saunders, 1976).

2. William Weiss et al., *American Review of Respiratory Disease* III: 289 (1975).

3. U. Veronesi et al., *New England Journal of Medicine,* 297 #12:627 (22 September 1977).

4. J. A. Del Regato, *Radiology* 88:761 (1967).

5. John Madden and S. Kandalaft, *Annals of Surgery,* 174:530 (1971). George Crile, Jr., and R. B. Turnbull, Jr., *Surgery, Gynecology and Obstetrics,* 135:1751–56 (September 1972).

6. J. R. Stjernsward et al., *Lancet,* 1352 (24 June 1972).

Chapter IV

1. George Crile, Jr., *Surgery, Gynecology and Obstetrics,* 83:-150–62 (August 1948).

2. M. L. Murphy et al., *New England Journal of Medicine* 297 #12:621 (22 September 1977).

3. Editorial, *New England Journal of Medicine,* 297 #12:661 (22 September 1977).

NOTES

Chapter V

1. Richard Spark, *New York Times Magazine* (25 July 1976), p. 10.
2. W. Weiss, H. Seidman, and K. R. Boucot, *American Review of Respiratory Disease,* III:289 (1975).

PART TWO

Chapter VI

1. Paper read at district meeting of Hospital Administrators of New England and New York State, Hartford, Conn., (12 May 1972).
2. J. H. Lavin and L. C. Busek, "What Makes Americans So Operation-Happy?" *Medical Economics* 50:67–75 (1973).
3. P. A. Lembeke, *American Journal of Public Health* 42:276–86 (1952).
4. George Rosemond, *Ca* 23:33 (January–February 1973).

Chapter VIII

1. *Bulletin of the American College of Surgeons* (November 1976), p. 22.
2. George Crile, Jr., "A Way to Identify Inappropriate Surgery," *American Medical News,* (16 February 1976).

Chapter IX

1. Presented at meeting of American Heart Association, (1974).

Chapter X

1. Eric J. Cassell, *The Healer's Art* (Philadelphia: J. B. Lippincott, 1976).
2. R. W. Cheadle, *American Medical News,* (22 November 1976), p. 5.

Notes

Chapter XI

1. D. G. Cullen et al., *New England Journal of Medicine*, 18: 982–987 (1976).

2. B. D. Colen, *Washington Post*, (22 July 1977).

3. Saul Kent, *Modern Medicine*, (1 February 1976), p. 54.

4. John Knowles, in *Doing Better and Feeling Worse: Health in the United States*, vol. 106, no. 1, of the Proceedings of the American Academy of Arts and Sciences (Winter 1977).

Index

Abdomen, annual examination of, 105
Abdominoperineal resection, 53, 54–55, 57–58
Adenoidectomy, 98
Adenomas, 77–81
Adrenal glands, 27–29
Adrenalectomy, medical, 28
Albert Einstein College of Medicine, 18
AMA News, 148
American Board of Surgery, 20
American Cancer Society, 8
American College of Surgeons, 139, 153, 157
American Heart Association, 142
American Hospital Association, 139
American Medical Association, 121, 136, 139, 148–149
American Surgical Association, 157
Anemia, 109
Anesthesiologists, 5
Aneurysm, 100
Angina pectoris, 82
Annual physical examination, value of, 102–109
Anterior resection, 52, 54
Antibiotics, 4, 5, 158
Antiestrogens, 28
Antrectomy and vagotomy, 72, 73

INDEX

Aorta, 100
Appendectomy, 120, 124, 134
Appendicitis, 66–67, 119–120
Arthritis, 67–68
Aspiration biopsy, 10, 13, 80, 81, 120–122
Axillary dissection, 14, 22, 23

Back pain, 68–69
Benign hypertrophy, 95
Beth Israel Hospital, 18
Biopsy, 10–13, 80, 81, 120–122
Blood counts, 109
Blood pressure, 107
Blood sugar level, 108
Blood tests, 154
Blue Cross, 135, 158
Blue Shield, 118–119, 134–135
Bonadonna, Dr., 28–29
Bone cancer, 108
Bone scans, 30
Bowel, cancer of, 107
Breast, The (Cope), 19–20
Breast cancer, 8–32, 144; biopsy, 10–13, 80, 81, 120–121; chemotherapy, 28–29, 65; choosing treatment, 31–32; differing opinions about treatment of, 8, 113–114; endocrine therapy, 25–28; mammography, 9–10, 106; radiation therapy, 14, 15, 16, 19–20, 24–25, 64; scans, 30; surgery, 13–24
"Breast Cancer: A Report to the Profession," 8
Breasts, examination of, 106
Bulletin of the American College of Surgeons, 135
Bunker, J. P., 119

Cancer: adjuncts to surgery, value of, 64–65; bone, 108; bowel, 107; breast. *See* Breast cancer; cervix, 34–37, 106; head, 37, 38; larynx, 39–41, 104; lung, 41–43, 105; melanomas, 43–45; metastases, 5; morbidity, 6; mouth, 38, 104; neck, 4, 37–38; nose, 104; ovaries, 106; pancreas, 46–47, 143, 157; prostate, 48–52, 97; rectum, 4, 52–58, 106, 137, 157; skin, 59–60; thyroid, 60–64, 77, 78–79; uterus, 106
Carlyon, W. M., 148
Carter, Tim Lee, 148
Cataracts, 103
Cauterization, 34, 35
Cervix, cancer of, 34–37, 106
Cheadle, R. W., 148
Checkups, value of, 102–109
Chemotherapy, 64, 65; breast cancer, 28–29, 65; skin cancer, 59, 60
Cholecystectomy, 73–76
Chondritis, 41
Chronic appendicitis, 66–67
Cimetidine, 70
Cleveland Academy of Medicine, Ethics Committee of, 121
Cleveland Clinic, 18, 46, 56–57, 63–64, 80, 82, 129
Cleveland Press, 149
Colon, polyps in, 93–94
Colostomy, 53, 56, 58
Complete physical examination, value of, 102–108
Conflict of interest, 115–118, 124, 125
Conization, 34, 35

[170]

INDEX

Consent, informed, 141–145
Contingency fee, 155
Controversy in Surgery (Varco and Delaney), 33
Cope, Oliver, 19–20
Coronary bypass surgery, 82–83, 142
Crile, George, Sr., 38
Cryotherapy, 34, 35, 59, 60, 114
Cysts: needle aspiration of, 10, 13, 121–122; pilonidal, 90–93; sebaceous, 90
Cytology, 5

Davis, Neville, 44
Delaney, J. P., 33
Detached retina, 103
Diabetes, 108
Diminishing returns, law of, 151–161
Direct inguinal hernia, 85
Dunlop, George R., 153, 154
Duodenal ulcer, 69–73

Ears, annual examination of, 104
Electrocardiograms, 107–108
Electrocoagulation, 54–58, 114
Electrosurgery, 59, 60
Endocrine therapy: breast cancer, 25–28; prostate cancer, 50, 52
England, 154–155
Esselstyn, C. B., Sr., 118–119
Estrogen, 27–28, 37, 50
Eyes, annual examination of, 103–104

Fee-for-service surgery, 113–126; benefits of, 127–128; conflict of interest and, 115–118, 124, 125; differing opinions about treatment and, 113–115; effect of fee size on operation selected, 120–122; effect of remuneration method on incidence of operations, 118–120; hospitals and, 125–126; inappropriate operations and, 134, 135; versus prepaid health plans, 127, 128, 130–131; referrals and, 115, 122–125; versus socialized practice, 128–130
Fibrositis, 67
Fisher, Bernard, 15, 21
Fitzpatrick, P. J., 26
Fox, M. S., 24
Frozen section, 10
Functionlust, 132–133

Gallstones, 73–76, 114, 137
Gastric resection, 71
Gastroenterostomy, 70; and vagotomy, 71
Genitalia, annual examination of, 105–106
Glaucoma, 103
Goiter, 76–81, 86–87
Graves' disease, 87–89

Halsted radical mastectomy, 4, 17, 19
Head, cancer of, 37, 38
Health care: law of diminishing returns and, 151–161; public education about, 146–150, 160–161
Health maintenance organization (HMO), 127, 128, 130–131

INDEX

Heart, annual examination of, 107–108
Heart disease, 82–83, 107, 157
Heart surgery, 138, 146
Heller, Joseph, 149–150
Hemorrhoidectomy, 83, 84
Hemorrhoids, 83–84
Hernia repair, 85–86, 124
Hip, replacement of, 67
Hormones: breast cancer and, 26–29; thyroid, 76–77, 79–80
Hospitals, 125–126, 159
Hyperthyroidism, 86–89, 137–138
Hysterectomy, 34–36, 124, 144

Implants, breast, 16, 22, 23
Inappropriate operations, 132–140
Indirect inguinal hernia, 85–86
Informed consent, 141–145
Ingrown toenails, 89–90
Inguinal hernia, 85–86
In-situ cancer, 34–37
Intubation of the trachea, 5
Inward goiter, 87

Johns Hopkins Hospital, 17

Kaiser Foundation, 127, 128, 130
Kidney failure, 107, 108–109, 147
Knowles, John, 160

Laboratory tests, value of, 108–109, 158
Lahey Clinic, 129
Laryngectomy, 39, 40
Larynx, cancer of, 39–41, 104
Levene, Martin B., 20

Ligation, 100
Lip, cancer of, 59
Lipomas, 90
Liver failure, 108, 109
Liver scans, 30
Lobectomy, 42
Lorenz, Konrad, 132
Lumpectomy, 16, 19, 23, 24
Lungs: annual examination of, 105; cancer of, 41–43, 105

M. D. Anderson Cancer Center, 18
McPherson, K., 24
Madden, John, 56–57
Malpractice insurance, 153, 154–155
Mammography, 9–10, 106
Massachusetts General Hospital, 18, 80, 154
Mastectomy, 4, 13–16; modified radical, 13, 15–18, 21, 22, 120, 122; partial, 13, 14, 15, 18, 23, 120; radical, 13–15, 17–19, 22, 24, 120, 121, 122, 133; simple, 14, 21, 22, 23, 120, 122; subcutaneous, 17, 23; ultraradical, 13, 14, 22
Mayo Clinic, 17, 63, 129
Medicaid, 115, 140, 149, 154
Medical adrenalectomy, 28
Medical Economics, 119
Medicare, 115, 128, 140, 149
Melanomas, 43–45
Memorial Hospital, New York, 80
Menopause, 36–37
Metastases, 5
Modified radical mastectomy, 13, 15–18, 21, 22, 120, 122

INDEX

Modified radical neck dissection, 38, 62
Morbidity, 6, 7
Mouth, cancer of, 38, 104

National Cancer Institute, 8, 15–16, 21, 28
National Institutes of Health, 9
National insurance program, 153
National Surgical Adjuvant Breast Project, 21
Neck: annual examination of, 104–105; cancer of, 4, 37–38; thyroid cancer caused by radiation treatment, 60, 62–64
Needle biopsy, 10, 13, 80, 81, 120–122
Nervous system, examination of, 107
New England Journal of Medicine, 44
New York Times, The, 136
Nipple transplant, 16–17, 23
Nixon, Richard M., 148
Node dissection, 43–45
Nodules, thyroid, 76–81
Nonpenetrating radiation, 53–54, 55, 58
Nose: annual examination of, 104; cancer of, 104

Ochsner Clinic, 129
Open biopsy, 11, 13, 120
Operations: effect of fee size on type of, 120–122; effect of remuneration method on incidence of, 118–120; inappropriate, 132–140; informed consent and, 141–145; *See also* specific operations

Otolaryngologists, 97
Ovaries: breast cancer and, 26–29, 36, 37; cancer of, 106
Overholt, Richard, 42

Paige, Satchel, 160
Pancreas, cancer of, 46–47, 143, 157
Pancreaticoduodenectomy, 46, 47
Papanicolaou test (Pap smear), 5, 6, 34, 106
Papillary cancers, 60–64, 78–79
Papillon, Jean, 54
Parathyroid glands, 108, 109
Partial laryngectomy, 39, 40
Partial mastectomy, 13, 14, 15, 18, 23, 120
Physical examination, value of, 102–109
Pierrequin, Dr., 24–25
Pilonidal cysts or sinuses, 90–93
Pituitary glands, 27–29
Polyps, 93–94
Prednisone, 28
Prepaid health plans, 118, 127, 128, 130–131
Presacral dermoid cysts, 93
President's Committee on Health Education, 148
Princess Margaret Hospital, 26
Proctoscopic examination, 107
Prolapse, 98
Prostate gland: benign enlargement of, 95–97; cancer of, 48–52, 97
Prostatectomy: radical, 49–50, 52; suprapubic, 96
Public education about health, 146–150, 160–161

[173]

INDEX

Pull-thru operation, 53, 54, 58
Pyloroplasty, 70; and vagotomy, 71, 73

Radiation: mammography and, 9–10; scans and, 30; thyroid cancer induced by, 60, 62–64
Radiation therapy, 114, 146–147; breast cancer, 14, 15, 16, 19–20, 24–25, 64; laryngeal cancer, 40; need for, 64–65; prostate cancer, 50–51, 52; rectal cancer, 53–54, 55, 58; skin cancer, 59, 60
Radical mastectomy, 13–15, 17–19, 21, 22, 24, 120, 121, 133
Radical neck dissection, 37–38, 62
Radical pancreaticoduodenectomy, 46–47
Radical prostatectomy, 49–50, 52
Radioactive iodine, 87–89, 137–138
Rectum: annual examination of, 106; cancer of, 4, 52–58, 106, 137, 157
Referrals, 115, 122–125
Relaxed inguinal ring, 85
Retinas, detached, 103
Richter, M. A., 142
Rosemond, George, 121
Rubber-band technique of hemorrhoidectomy, 84
Ruptured discs, 68

San Diego Naval Hospital, 92
Sandburg, Helga, 69
Scans, 30
Sebaceous cysts, 90

Selective vagotomy, 72, 73
Sequential multiple analyses, 108, 109
Shaw, George Bernard, 116
Shouldice Clinic, 86
Simple mastectomy, 14, 21, 22, 23, 120, 122
Skin, cancers of, 59–60
Skin graft, 59, 60
Socialized practice, 128–130
Spark, Richard, 102
Specialists, 123
Stjernsward, J. R., 64
Strauss, Abraham, 56
Stricture, 83, 84
Stripping, 100
Strokes, 101
Subcutaneous mastectomy, 17, 23
Subtotal gastrectomy, 71
Sulfanilamide, 4
Suprapubic prostatectomy, 96
Sympathectomy, 135
Syphilis, 109

Tamoxifen, 28
Tetany, thyroidectomy and, 63, 83
Throat, annual examination of, 104
Thromboses, 99
Thyroid gland: cancer of, 60–64, 77, 78–79; goiter, 76–81, 86–87; hyperthyroidism, 86–89, 137–138
Thyroidectomy, 63, 81, 89, 137
Thyroid-stimulating hormone, 76–77
Thyroiditis, 137
Tissue committee, 139
Toenails, ingrown, 89–90

INDEX

Tongue, cancer of, 38
Tonsilectomy, 97–98, 134, 136
Trachea, intubation of, 5
Transurethral resection, 50, 51, 52, 96
Tuberculosis, 105
Tylectomy, 24

Ulcer, duodenal, 69–73
Ultraradical mastectomy, 13, 14, 22
University of Toronto, Princess Margaret Hospital, 18
Uterus: cancer of, 106; hysterectomy, 34–36, 124, 144; prolapse of, 98; suspension of, 134, 135

Vaginal repair operations, 98–99
Vagotomy, 71; and antrectomy, 72, 73; and gastroenterostomy, 71; and pyloroplasty, 71, 73; selective, 72, 73
Varco, R. L., 33
Varicose veins, 99–100; hemorrhoids, 83–84
Vascular surgery, 100–101
Veterans Administration Hospitals, 54, 83
Vision, loss of, 103–104
Vocal cords: cancer of, 39; radioactive iodine therapy and, 87, 88

Wassink, W. F., 56
Wens, 90
Whipple, Allen, 46
White, Ken L., 119
World Health Organization, 44

Yale University Medical School, 18

The Author

George Crile, Jr., M.D., is Emeritus Consultant in Surgery at the Cleveland Clinic and an internationally recognized authority on treatment of breast cancer and thyroid disease. He is the author of many books, both for professionals and for the lay reader, including *Cancer and Common Sense, A Naturalistic View of Man,* and *What Women Should Know About the Breast Cancer Controversy.*